Meet the editor

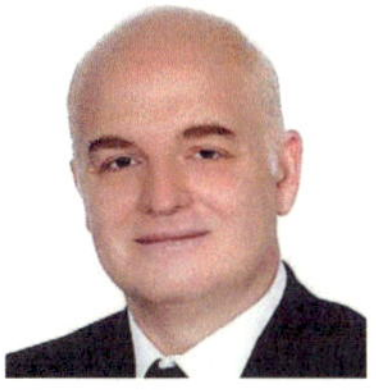

Dr. Ahmet Mesrur Halefoğlu is currently a resident specialist in Radiology and a Professor at Sisli Etfal Training and Research Hospital in Istanbul, Turkey. He completed Antakya High School in Antakya, Hatay, Turkey, with honors, and graduated from Istanbul University Cerrahpaşa School of Medicine in 1986, Istanbul, Turkey. He completed his residency from 1992 to 1997 at Sisli Etfal Training and Research Hospital in İstanbul, Turkey. He served as a postdoctoral research fellow at Johns Hopkins Hospital in Baltimore, MD, USA, from 1998 to 1999. He has also been a Research Observer at Johns Hopkins Hospital in 2002 and 2004. He primarily works in body imaging and neuroradiology, using multi-detector computed tomography and high-resolution magnetic resonance imaging. He has more than 60 high-impact factor publications and has written 3 book chapters. He is a member of the Turkish Society of Radiology and the European Society of Radiology.

Contents

Preface

It is my honor to introduce the book entitled *Computed Tomography - An Overview*.

Computed tomography (CT) remains a cornerstone of contemporary diagnostic imaging, providing high-resolution anatomical and functional information essential for clinical decision-making. As technological advancements accelerate, a concise yet authoritative overview of CT has become increasingly important for practitioners and trainees. *Computed Tomography - An Overview* was developed to address this need by presenting fundamental principles and current innovations within a coherent, academically structured framework.

CT plays a pivotal role across a wide range of clinical disciplines, including emergency medicine, oncology, cardiovascular imaging, and interventional planning. Its rapid acquisition, superior spatial resolution, and ability to characterize tissues render it indispensable in the evaluation of acute conditions such as trauma, stroke, pulmonary embolism, and abdominal emergencies. In oncology, CT remains central to staging, assessment of treatment response, and long-term surveillance. At the same time, advances in cardiac imaging have expanded its utility for coronary artery evaluation and procedural planning. These broad applications underscore CT's centrality in modern patient management and highlight the need for optimized techniques and evidence-based interpretation.

I hope that this book will serve as a reliable reference for radiologists, residents, and all professionals engaged in medical imaging, supporting both academic study and informed clinical practice.

Ahmet Mesrur Halefoglu, M.D.
Department of Radiology,
Sisli Hamidiye Etfal Training and Research Hospital,
Istanbul, Turkey

Chapter 1

Introductory Chapter: Computed Tomography in Modern Radiology Practice

Ahmet Mesrur Halefoglu

1. Introduction

Computed tomography (CT) is an imaging modality that produces cross-sectional images of the human body via X-rays. Its first clinical use started in the early 1970s after being developed by Godfrey Hounsfield [1]. It has since become one of the most essential imaging tools, with various clinical applications including emergency trauma cases, neurology, cardiology, and oncology fields. CT has important advantages in terms of providing high-resolution, detailed anatomical images in short time periods [2]. The main advantage of CT over plain film radiography is its ability to generate cross-sectional axial plane images and also to produce reconstructed images in sagittal and coronal planes, thus providing good-quality multiplanar body images.

2. Technical features

The basic principle of CT is based on the measurement of X-ray attenuation of tissues. The collected data obtained from the attenuation values of the examined body region are processed by a computer system, and thus, axial plane cross-sectional images are created. These images can also be reconstructed in sagittal and coronal planes, and even in three-dimensional (3D) format [2]. The CT system consists of a gantry, which may be in a ring or cylinder fashion, into which a patient is placed. The X-ray tube and X-ray detector spin rapidly in the gantry as the patient is moved in and out of the gantry. Multi-detector CT (MDCT) scanners provide more rapid image acquisition and better image spatial resolution compared to those of single-slice CT systems [3]. Computer software is used for image processing, volumetric reconstruction, and 3D modeling [2]. The image quality depends on several parameters, including tube voltage (kVp), tube current (mA), slice thickness, pixel resolution, and matrix size. Besides, the use of orally or intravenously administered contrast agents enhances tissue differentiation, but motion artifacts due to patient movement or respiration can cause image degradation [2, 3].

IntechOpen

3. Clinical applications

CT has a wide spectrum of clinical applications. In the neurology field, it is crucial to get a rapid assessment of head trauma, hemorrhage, stroke, and also the evaluation of brain tumors and vascular malformations [4]. In the thorax, it provides a comprehensive evaluation of mediastinal lesions, pulmonary nodules and masses, and pulmonary embolism [5]. In the abdomen and pelvis, it reveals pathologies of the liver, pancreas, spleen, kidney, adrenal glands, gallbladder, and urinary bladder, and can also be used for trauma evaluation [2]. In orthopedics, bone fractures, joint, and soft tissue pathologies can be demonstrated. In the oncology field, CT has a crucial role and enables tumor detection, localization, staging, treatment planning, and follow-up [2, 4]. In the cardiology field, coronary artery CT angiography provides a noninvasive evaluation of coronary arteries [4]. The CT has diverse clinical indications, especially when rapid, high-quality images are necessary. It provides rapid diagnosis in emergency situations like stroke, trauma, internal bleeding, and obstruction [4]. It is also valuable in the detection of suspected tumors or metastases and the evaluation of bone, soft tissue, and joint injuries. It also has diagnostic capability in lung diseases like pneumonia and pulmonary embolism. CT plays an important role in the diagnosis of abdominal and pelvic diseases like cirrhosis, pancreatitis, stones, inflammatory bowel disease, and pelvic disease. It can also be used for noninvasive coronary artery disease evaluation by coronary CT angiography [4].

4. Limitations and disadvantages

Despite its invaluable diagnostic value, CT has some limitations. One of the main concerns is radiation exposure, which leads to significant cumulative radiation in the general population [5, 6]. Therefore, it should be carefully performed, especially in children and young adult patients. Another limitation of CT is the possible risk associated with contrast agents, which can lead to allergic reactions, including anaphylaxis and nephrotoxicity [2].

Soft tissue limitation is another issue, and MRI has superiority compared to CT in terms of soft tissue contrast resolution.

Motion artifacts due to patient breathing and movement can cause image degradation. Finally, cost-effectiveness is a limitation because advanced CT techniques, like CT angiography, MDCT, and 3D reconstructions, may be too expensive [3]. CT is improving its diagnostic performance depending on ongoing technological advances. Low-dose CT protocols aim to reduce radiation exposure while providing good-quality images [4]. Artificial intelligence (AI) and deep learning algorithms are increasingly being integrated into CT systems and enable automated lesion detection and diagnostic support that enhance diagnostic performance. Functional CT techniques allow quantitative assessment of tissue perfusion and vascular dynamics. Hybrid imaging systems, such as positron emission tomography (PET)/CT, combine anatomical and metabolic information and improve diagnostic accuracy [2, 4].

5. Conclusion

In conclusion, CT is an excellent imaging modality that provides high spatial resolution and detailed anatomical images in a short scanning time. It is a highly accurate and reliable imaging modality and should be used appropriately in necessary conditions. However, radiation exposure and contrast agent-related risks must always be considered. CT protocols should always be consistent with the ALARA principle (As Low As Reasonably Achievable) [5, 6].

Author details

Ahmet Mesrur Halefoglu
University of Health Sciences Şişli Hamidiye Etfal Training and Research Hospital, Istanbul, Turkey

*Address all correspondence to: halefoglu@hotmail.com

References

[1] Hounsfield GN. Computerized transverse axial scanning (tomography): Part 1. Description of system. The British Journal of Radiology. 1973;**46**(552):1016–1022

[2] Kalender WA. Computed Tomography: Fundamentals, System Technology, Image Quality. Applications. 3rd ed. Weinheim, Germany: Wiley-VCH; 2011

[3] Mahesh M. MDCT Physics: The Basics – Technology, Image Quality and Radiation Dose. 2nd ed. Philadelphia, Pennsylvania, USA: Lippincott Williams & Wilkins; 2018

[4] McCollough CH, Chen GH, Kalender W, Leng S, Samei E, Taguchi K, Wang G, Lifeng Y, Pettigrewal RI. Achieving routine submillisievert CT scanning: Report from the summit on management of radiation dose in CT. Radiology. 2012;**264**(2):567–580

[5] Mayo JR, Aldrich J, Muller NI. Radiation exposure at chest CT: A statement of the Fleischner Society. Radiology. 2003;**228**(1):15–21

[6] Brenner DJ, Hall EJ. Computed tomography — An increasing source of radiation exposure. New England Journal of Medicine. 2007;**357**(22):2277–2284

Chapter 2

Patient Preparation for Computed Tomography

Khayyal Mohammed

Abstract

Proper patient preparation is essential for a safe and accurate computed tomography (CT) scan. Most practices require special preparation for non-emergency scans. Some special situations may require additional steps for preparation. This chapter will discuss different aspects of patient preparation for CT scan. These include patient education, dietary restriction, medication management, vascular access, positioning and shielding. In addition to that, there are several special situations that require additional preparatory considerations before CT scan. One of these special situations is performing CT coronary angiography. This special type of scan requeires heart rate control and administration of medications to cause coronary vasodilatation. Administration of iodinated contrast media is very frequently required with CT scans. This requires establishment of vascular access. Prior history of allergy to iodinated contrast media also requires special care. Special care also should be practiced in cases of kidney disease, thyroid disease, pregnant ladies and pediatric population. Patients at high risk of contrast inducedacute kidney injury require active preparation to lower the posiibility of development of such serious complication.

Keywords: patient preparation, pre-scan, medication, allergy, contrast-induced nephropathy

1. Introduction

Computed tomography (CT) is a widely used imaging modality. It is used in a wide range of medical conditions. While many types of CT scans can be readily done without special preparation, many CT scans require special preparations for safe and sound imaging results. In this chapter, we will cover patient preparation for CT scans.

2. Patient education and informed consent

Informed consent should be obtained from the patient or their legal guardian after a clear explanation of the procedure, its indications, and hazards. The preparation of printed leaflets explaining these aspects saves time and effort for the staff. Additionally, providing video clips with clear and suitable language to answer frequently asked questions is of great value and improves patient satisfaction [1]. Many institutions allow verbal consent for radiologic procedures involving contrast administration [2]. Due to the diversity in laws and policies regarding this issue, it is essential to review the laws of your locality, local guidelines, and departmental or hospital policies [3].

3. Dietary restrictions and fasting requirements

Most practices require a minimum duration of fasting for four to six hours before contrast-enhanced CT scans. This is historically claimed to reduce the risk of nausea and vomiting, with subsequent possible aspiration. Prolonged fasting is not just a cause of patient discomfort but also carries the risk of hypoglycemia in diabetic patients [3]. However, a study published in 2012 showed that the risk of aspiration does not increase with the ingestion of clear fluids before contrast-enhanced CT scans [4]. Another study confirmed similar findings in cancer patients in 2018 [5]. The necessity and rationality of fasting are increasingly questioned by clinical and radiology departments. Preparatory fasting may still give practitioners and policymakers a sense of security, even if false [6]. According to the recommendations of the American College of Radiology (ACR), preparatory fasting is not routinely recommended for non-gastrointestinal contrast-enhanced CT scans [3]. Fasting is still required if the CT scan requires sedation. The recommended fasting duration is two hours for clear fluids, six hours for a light meal, and eight hours for high-fat solids [7].

Caffeine may interfere with efforts to control heart rate before a cardiac CT scan or CT coronary angiography. Therefore, it is recommended to avoid caffeinated beverages for at least 12 hours before undergoing these scans [8].

Despite the lack of evidence in the literature regarding abstinence from smoking before a planned CT scan, some practices advise avoiding smoking for 24 hours before a contrast-enhanced CT scan.

4. Medication management

Some medications may have adverse interactions with iodinated contrast or increase its risks. Some special scans require preparation through the administration of certain medications. Here, we will discuss some common examples.

4.1 Metformin

Historically, metformin was suggested to be discontinued before the administration of iodinated contrast for fear of contrast-induced acute kidney injury (CI-AKI) [9]. However, metformin was not found to increase the risk of CI-AKI, but it was associated with an increased incidence of lactic acidosis in patients who develop CI-AKI [10]. The ACR does not recommend the discontinuation of metformin before the intravenous administration of iodinated contrast media if the patient does not have AKI and the estimated glomerular filtration rate (eGFR) is 30 mL/minute or more. If the eGFR is <30 mL/minute or iodinated contrast is going to be administered into the renal artery, it is advised to withhold metformin for 48 hours before the procedure [3].

4.2 Heart rate control in CT coronary angiography

Cardiac motion represents a major challenge and source of artifacts in cases of CT coronary angiography. To reduce the incidence of this artifact, heart rate needs to be controlled, with a target heart rate of 60 beats per minute (bpm). The first line of medications for controlling heart rate is oral beta-blockers, supplemented with IV beta-blockers at the time of the scan if the target heart rate is not achieved by oral beta-blockers. Patients with active bronchial asthma cannot tolerate beta-blockers, and other alternatives should be administered [11]. Be aware that beta-blockers may lower the threshold for contrast reactions. Additionally, they may blunt the effect of epinephrine in cases of anaphylaxis. However, due to the low incidence of anaphylaxis, beta-blockers can be given, which need not be stopped for any contrast-enhanced scan [3].

Ivabradine acts directly on the sinoatrial node by inhibition of the I_f current. Its use is recommended when beta-blockers cannot be used or cannot achieve heart rate control alone. However, oral administration of ivabradine must be started five days before the planned procedure to allow the effect of the drug to take place. Intravenous ivabradine can be used, but it is not widely available. Additionally, ivabradine cannot be used in cases of atrial fibrillation [8].

Non-dihydropyridine calcium channel blockers (verapamil and diltiazem) were attempted to be used for heart rate control during CT coronary angiography, but the results were not satisfactory. Their use for this purpose should be limited to cases where other agents have failed or are contraindicated [12].

4.3 Nephroprotective drugs

Prophylaxis for renal toxicity of contrast agents should be considered for patients with AKI or severe chronic kidney disease with an eGFR less than 30 mL/min/1.73 m^2 [3]. Hydration by infusion of intravenous normal saline is the only preventive measure that has shown a significant reduction in the nephrotoxic effects of iodinated contrast media in at-risk populations. Two different protocols can be used for intravenous hydration. The long protocol uses an intravenous infusion of 1 mL/kg 0.9% NaCl for 12 hours before the planned contrast-enhanced CT and continues for 12 hours after the procedure. The short protocol uses an infusion of 3–4 mL/kg 0.9% NaCl for four hours before and four hours after the planned procedure. Caution should be taken in cases with cardiovascular disease to monitor for signs and symptoms of lung congestion [13, 14]. A meta-analysis of six studies showed that oral hydration is not inferior to intravenous hydration in the prevention of contrast-induced nephropathy [15]. However, oral hydration has not yet been evaluated in high-risk patients [16]. The ENRICH trial is addressing this issue, but it is still in the recruitment phase [17].

N-acetylcysteine was historically used to reduce the risk of contrast-induced nephropathy [18, 19]. Pre-procedural administration of N-acetylcysteine did not show a reduction in the risk of CI-AKI [20].

Historically, several other drugs were suggested for renal prophylaxis against nephrotoxicity, for example, theophylline, sodium bicarbonate, prostaglandin E1, ascorbic acid, allopurinol, alpha-tocopherol, fenoldopam, and trimetazidine. No trials have shown clinical benefits of any of these medications, and the use of these medications is not recommended [21].

Also, prophylactic hemodialysis did not prevent CI-AKI after exposure to iodinated contrast media in at-risk patients [22].

4.4 Nephrotoxic drugs

It was advised that nephrotoxic drugs such as non-steroidal anti-inflammatory drugs (NSAIDs), aminoglycosides, vancomycin, and amphotericin B be withheld before the administration of iodinated contrast agents [18]. However, no specific recommendations were provided to stop these medications in the guidelines of the ACR or the Canadian Association of Radiologists [3, 21].

4.5 Allergic reaction prophylaxis

Incidence of allergic reactions to iodinated contrast media is estimated to be 0.6% for all reactions and about 0.04% for severe reactions. The risk of allergic reactions related to contrast media is higher in females and in the middle-aged population as compared with other population classes. Patients with previous non-contrast-related allergic reactions are at a two- to threefold increased risk of allergic reactions to contrast. Patients with prior contrast-related allergic reactions are at the greatest risk for recurrent allergic reactions if exposed to the same class of contrast media. Patients with bronchial asthma are more prone to allergic reactions that usually manifest with bronchospasm.

Patients with severe cardiovascular disease, such as severe aortic stenosis or advanced heart failure, do not exhibit an increased risk of allergic reactions per se but typically experience severe hemodynamic consequences if allergic reactions occur. This increased vulnerability usually manifests as more profound hypotension and pulmonary congestion. Additionally, if patients on beta-blockers develop anaphylaxis, their response to injected epinephrine can be blunted [3].

Intradermal skin testing before the administration of contrast media has not been shown to be useful [23]. The premedication protocol has demonstrated benefits in reducing the incidence and severity of allergic-like reactions related to contrast media. However, premedication does not guarantee the prevention of severe allergic reactions, and the team must be prepared to manage such reactions if they occur. Premedication is only indicated for patients with a previous allergic reaction to iodinated contrast media. Patients with other allergies, such as allergies to shell-fish or povidone-iodine, are not indicated for premedication.

The preferred premedication protocol is by oral administration of 50 mg of oral prednisone at 13, 7, and 1 hour(s) before the planned procedure, with 50 mg of oral diphenhydramine 1 hour before the procedure. An accelerated intravenous protocol can be used as an alternative by administration of 50 mg intravenous (IV) diphenhydramine 1 hour before the scan and either 200 mg of IV hydrocortisone or 40 mg IV methylprednisolone 4 – 5 hours before the scan [3, 24, 25].

5. Vascular access

For the injection of contrast agents, vascular access must be established. The vascular access may vary according to the type of scan required. Usually, peripheral intravenous access is achieved using a flexible plastic cannula. The use of metal needles should be avoided. The preferred site of injection is the antecubital or a large forearm vein. A 22-gauge catheter can tolerate flow rates up to 5 mL/s; however, a larger-sized catheter is preferred. The use of power injectors is generally recommended. Careful preparation of the power injector device is mandatory to avoid air embolism and extravasation [3]. The risk of extravasation is lowest if an upper arm vein is used for injection compared with other locations [26]. The use of external jugular veins for the administration of contrast media is not recommended due to the high risk of extravasation [27].

In general, a central venous catheter can be used for the administration of contrast media, but the assumption that power injection can be performed in all central venous catheters should not be made. For a central line to be used for power injection of contrast media, it must be tested to withstand a pressure of 300 psi or greater [3, 27]. Before the use of a central venous catheter for contrast administration, the back flow of blood should be tested, as well as the resistance to saline injection. If abnormally high resistance is found, alternative access should be established.

If the establishment of intravenous access is not possible, intra-osseous injection can be used. However, the injection rate and pressure settings have not been widely studied [3].

6. Patient exposure, positioning and shielding

Although most CT scans can be done without the need for special clothing for the patient, many institutions still require the patient to change into special garments like hospital gowns. A balance between patient comfort, dignity, safety, and scan quality must be achieved. Metallic objects (like jewelry and zippers) must be avoided in the scan field. Clothing must not interfere with proper positioning, alignment, and access to the IV line for contrast administration [28].

Optimal positioning for CT scans should guarantee patient safety and comfort, as well as the best image quality. Most CT scans are done in the supine position. The patient must be positioned in the center of the gantry for the best image quality and reduced radiation exposure. The use of support or immobilization devices is essential to maintain patient comfort and avoid motion artifacts [29].

In cases of head CT, the head is kept in a neutral position with anatomical landmarks aligned parallel to the scanning plane. The aim is to achieve image symmetry to facilitate interpretation. In cases of CT chest or cardiac CT, the arms are placed above the head to keep them away from the scan field and to avoid beam hardening artifacts [30]. In cases of CT abdomen and pelvis, the patient usually lies supine with knees supported for comfort. Artificial intelligence-based patient positioning was more accurate in computed tomography of kidneys, ureters and bladder (KUB CT), resulting in less radiation exposure and better image quality [31].

Use of radioprotective material (usually lead or bismuth) for shielding to protect superficial radiosensitive organs may be considered. The most commonly shielded organs are the gonads, breasts, thyroid, and eyes [32, 33, 34]. However, shielding has some disadvantages. It may result in a reduction in image quality. Also, it may result in an increase in the total dose of patient radiation, especially if the tube current modulation function is used [35].

7. Special situations

7.1 Claustrophobia and anxiety

Patient anxiety and claustrophobia are well-known problems faced during magnetic resonance imaging (MRI). CT is usually thought of as an alternative to MRI in such cases. However, claustrophobia is still a serious problem in CT scans, despite being less frequent than it is in MRI. Claustrophobia can result in patient restlessness and motion artifacts, with subsequent degradation of image quality. Anxiety is more common in females, older patients, and in patients without prior CT scans [36, 37]. Additionally, anxiety may increase heart rate and affect the quality of CT coronary angiography [38]. Patient education has been helpful in reducing anxiety scores and improving patient satisfaction during CT scans [39]. Benzodiazepines can be administered prior to the test to alleviate anxiety in cumbersome cases [38].

7.2 Pediatric patients

Careful patient assessment before a CT scan is of utmost importance in pediatric patients. The proper indication for a CT scan must be reviewed. Due to higher lifelong radiation exposure in pediatric patients, CT scans are better avoided if a reasonable alternative, like MRI, is available. In cases where a CT scan is the only option, the use of radiation reduction protocols must be emphasized. Careful pre-scan assessment is also required regarding patient cooperation and the possible need for sedation [40]. The use of a fast scan protocol can eliminate the need for anesthesia while preserving the quality of CT scans [41].

If the injection of contrast media is needed, an intravenous line should be inserted before the patient arrives at the radiology department to reduce patient agitation at the scanner [40]. Proper patient positioning at the isocenter of the gantry helps to achieve better image quality as well as reduces the radiation dose. The use of laser beams on the scanner is most useful in this regard [42].

7.3 Pregnancy and breast feeding

Elective CT scans are generally avoided during pregnancy due to the risks of radiation exposure to the fetus. However, the increasing utilization of CT scans in emergency settings has raised the issue of the use of CT scans in pregnant women. In general, most practitioners try to avoid CT scans during pregnancy and replace them with ultrasound scans or magnetic resonance imaging. However, a CT scan may remain the only or the last resort in some cases [43].

Routine screening for pregnancy is routinely conducted in many institutions before exposure to any procedure involving ionizing radiation. However, the ACR only requires screening for pregnancy in scans involving the region of the abdomen and pelvis, as well as nuclear scans. Screening for pregnancy includes history-taking as well as blood tests for beta-hCG levels, if necessary [44].

When the fetus is out of the field of view, the radiation dose received by the fetus is negligible. For example, the fetal radiation dose in a CT chest is 0.2 mGy or less, depending on the trimester. Routine CT of the abdomen and pelvis results in fetal radiation exposure of 25 mGy. With recently modified protocols for lowering fetal radiation exposure, CT of the abdomen and pelvis can be done with fetal exposure of 10–11 mGy. Shielding of the gravid uterus has shown little or no benefit in the reduction of fetal exposure to radiation [45].

Pregnancy outcome is not affected if maternal exposure to radiation is less than 500 mGy during pregnancy. However, a fetal radiation dose of 100 mGy results in a 0.1% increase in the risk of childhood cancer. The application of the As Low As Reasonably Achievable (ALARA) principle is most stressed in these situations [43].

Iodinated contrast media are known to cross the blood–placental barrier. A concern about neonatal affection of thyroid function was raised after exposure to iodinated contrast media, but studies have shown no effect on neonatal thyroid-stimulating hormone. No specific screening for pregnancy is indicated before the administration of iodinated contrast media. Most iodinated contrast media are classified as pregnancy category B by the FDA [3].

Absorption of iodinated contrast media from an infant's intestine is very low. So, there is no need to stop breast-feeding for lactating mothers who receive iodinated contrast media [3].

7.4 Implanted devices

The incidence of patients with implanted devices is increasing in the current era. Although it is generally safe to perform CT scans in most of these patients without specific preparations, certain situations can arise with such patients. In cases involving permanent cardiac pacemakers, exposure of the device to CT radiation results in increased sensing by the device. This may lead to temporary pacemaker malfunction. However, due to the short duration of most CT scans, this usually does not have a clinical impact on the patient [46]. If a patient with a cardiac pacemaker is undergoing CT coronary angiography, the pacemaker must be programmed to a set rate lower than 65 bpm before the scan. If the intrinsic patient rate is higher than that, the administration of beta-blockers is advised. It is worth mentioning that pacemaker and ICD leads result in significant artifacts in CT coronary angiography [47].

CT scans, in the presence of implanted devices such as neurostimulators, cochlear implants, and drug delivery pumps, are considered safe and require no specific precautions or preparations [48–50].

7.5 Thyroid disease

Administration of iodinated contrast media may potentiate thyrotoxicosis in known thyrotoxic patients. Thus, administration of iodinated contrast media should be avoided in acute thyrotoxicosis to prevent thyroid storm [51]. Additionally, iodinated contrast media should not be administered to patients with planned radioactive iodine administration for imaging or therapeutic purposes. If iodinated contrast media is administered in such patients, a wash-out period must be observed before the administration of radioactive iodine. The wash-out period should be three to four weeks for patients with hyperthyroidism and six weeks for hypothyroid patients [52].

7.6 Myasthenia gravis

Myasthenia gravis was considered a relative contraindication to the administration of iodinated intravenous contrast. A retrospective study showed delayed exacerbation of myasthenic symptoms in 6% of patients after exposure to iodinated contrast media [53]. However, given that the evidence comes only from a single retrospective study, no clear recommendations have been issued regarding this concern yet [3].

Author details

Khayyal Mohammed
Mansoura Health Insurance Hospital, Mansoura, Egypt

*Address all correspondence to: dr_m_khayyal@hotmail.com

References

[1] Sahai A, Kucheria R, Challacombe B, Dasgupta P. Video consent: A pilot study of informed consent in laparoscopic urology and its impact on patient satisfaction. JSLS. 2006;**10**(1):21–5

[2] Hadley LC, Watson T. The radiographers' role in information giving prior to consent for computed tomography scans: A cross-sectional survey. Radiography. 2016;**22**(4):e252–7

[3] ACR. Manual on contrast media 2025 ACR committee on drugs and contrast media. 2025

[4] Lee BY, Ok JJ, Elsayed AAA, Kim Y, Han DH. Preparative fasting for contrast-enhanced CT: Reconsideration. Radiology. 2012;**263**(2):444–450

[5] Barbosa PNVP, Bitencourt AGV, Tyng CJ, Cunha R, Travesso DJ, Almeida MFA, et al. Preparative fasting for contrast-enhanced CT in a cancer center: A new approach. American Journal of Roentgenology. 2018;**210**:941–947

[6] Liu H, Liu Y, Zhao L, Li X, Zhang W. Preprocedural fasting for contrast-enhanced CT: When experience meets evidence. Insights into Imaging. 2021;**12**:180

[7] Practice guidelines for preoperative fasting and the use of pharmacologic agents to reduce the risk of pulmonary aspiration: Application to healthy patients undergoing elective procedures. Anesthesiology. 2017, **126**(3):376–393

[8] Abbara S, Blanke P, Maroules CD, Cheezum M, Choi AD, Han BK, et al. SCCT guidelines for the performance and acquisition of coronary computed tomographic angiography: A report of the society of cardiovascular computed tomography guidelines committee: Endorsed by the North American Society for Cardiovascular Imaging (NASCI). Journal of Cardiovascular Computed Tomography. 2016;**10**:435–449

[9] Baerlocher MO, Asch M, Myers A. Metformin and intravenous contrast. CMAJ Canadian Medical Association Journal. 2013;**185**(1):E78

[10] Kao TW, Lee KH, Chan WP, Fan KC, Liu CW, Huang YC. Continuous use of metformin in patients receiving contrast medium: What is the evidence? A systematic review and meta-analysis. European Radiology. 2022;**32**(5):3045–3055

[11] Mahabadi AA, Achenbach S, Burgstahler C, Dill T, Fischbach R, Knez A, et al. Safety, efficacy, and indications of β-adrenergic receptor blockade to reduce heart rate prior to coronary CT angiography. Radiology. 2010;**257**:614–623

[12] Rogowski S, Lesslie VW, Ebersberger U. Drugs in Cardiac CT. In Schoepf UJ, editor. CT of the Heart. Totowa, NJ: Humana Press; 2019. p. 103–107. Available from: 10.1007/978-1-60327-237-7_9

[13] Nijssen EC, Rennenberg RJ, Nelemans PJ, Essers BA, Janssen MM, Vermeeren MA, et al. Prophylactic hydration to protect renal function from intravascular iodinated contrast material in patients at high risk of contrast-induced nephropathy

(AMACING): A prospective, randomised, phase 3, controlled, open-label, non-inferiority trial. The Lancet. 2017;**389**:1312–1322

[14] Nijssen EC, Nelemans PJ, Rennenberg RJ, Theunissen RA, van Ommen V, Wildberger JE. Prophylaxis in high-risk patients with eGFR < 30 mL/min/1.73 m2: Get the balance right. Investigative Radiology. 2019;**54** (9):580–588

[15] Cheungpasitporn W, Thongprayoon C, Brabec BA, Edmonds PJ, O′ Corragain OA, Erickson SB. Oral hydration for prevention of contrast-induced acute kidney injury in elective radiological procedures: A systematic review and meta-analysis of randomized controlled trials. North American Journal of Medical Sciences. 2014;**6**(12):618–624

[16] Davenport MS, Perazella MA, Yee J, Dillman JR, Fine D, McDonald RJ, et al. Use of intravenous iodinated contrast media in patients with kidney disease: Consensus statements from the American College of Radiology and the National Kidney Foundation. Radiology. 2020;**294**:660–668

[17] Clinicaltrials. Available from: https://clinicaltrials.gov/study/NCT05283512 [Accessed: 2025-September-16]

[18] Andreucci M, Faga T, Pisani A, Sabbatini M, Russo D, Michael A. Prevention of contrast-induced nephropathy through a knowledge of its pathogenesis and risk factors. The Scientific World Journal. 2014;**2014**:823169

[19] Widmark JM. Imaging-Related medications: A class overview. Baylor University Medical Center Proceedings. 2007;**20**(4):408–417

[20] Weisbord SD, Gallagher M, Jneid H, Garcia S, Cass A, Thwin SS, et al. Outcomes after Angiography with Sodium Bicarbonate and Acetylcysteine. New England Journal of Medicine. 2018;**378**:603–614

[21] Macdonald DB, Hurrell C, Costa AF, McInnes MDF, O'Malley ME, Barrett B, et al. Canadian association of radiologists guidance on contrast associated acute kidney injury. Canadian Association of Radiologists Journal. 2022;**73**:499–514

[22] Kawashima S, Takano H, Iino Y, Takayama M, Takano T. Prophylactic hemodialysis does not prevent contrast-induced nephropathy after cardiac catheterization in patients with chronic renal insufficiency. Circulation Journal. 2006;**70**(5):553–558

[23] Trcka J, Schmidt C, Seitz CS, Bröcker EB, Gross GE, Trautmann A. Anaphylaxis to iodinated contrast material: Nonallergic hypersensitivity or IgE-mediated allergy? American Journal of Roentgenology. 2008;**190** (3):666–670

[24] Chiu TM, Chu SY. Hypersensitivity reactions to iodinated contrast media. Biomedicine. 2022;**10**:1036

[25] Kang HR, Jeong J, Brockow K. Diagnosis and prevention of hypersensitivity reactions to iodinated contrast media. Allergy, Asthma and Immunology Research. Korean Academy of Asthma, Allergy and Clinical Immunology. 2022;**14**:348–360

[26] Stowell JR, Rigdon D, Colglazier R, Filler L, Orosco D, Connell M, et al. Risk of contrast extravasation with vascular access in computed tomography. Emergency

Radiology. 2020;**27**(3):253–258. DOI: 10.1007/s10140-020-01752-x

[27] Earhart A, McMahon P. Vascular access and contrast media. Journal of Infusion Nursing. 2011;**34**(2):97–105

[28] Yh C, Choi J, Han S. Functional and safety considerations in patient clothes during pandemic An infodemiological network analysis and LDA topic modeling. The Research Journal of the Costume Culture. 2024;**32**(5):636–652

[29] Al-Hayek Y, Zheng X, Hayre C, Spuur K. The influence of patient positioning on radiation dose in CT imaging: A narrative review. Journal of Medical Imaging and Radiation Sciences. 2022;**53**(4):737–747. DOI: 10.1016/j.jmir.2022.09.027

[30] Kazerooni EA, Austin JHM, Black WC, Dyer DS, Hazelton TR, Leung AN, et al. ACR–STR Practice Parameter for the Performance and Reporting of Lung Cancer Screening Thoracic Computed Tomography (CT): 2014 (Resolution 4)* Journal of Thoracic Imaging. 2014;**29**(5):310–316. DOI: 10.1097/RTI.0000000000000097

[31] Kundu S, Nayak K, Kadavigere R, Pendem S. Evaluation of positioning accuracy, radiation dose and image quality: Artificial intelligence based automatic versus manual positioning for CT KUB. F1000Research. 2024;**13**:683

[32] Karim MKA, Rahim NA, Matsubara K, Hashim S, Mhareb MHA, Musa Y. The effectiveness of bismuth breast shielding with protocol optimization in CT Thorax examination. Journal of X-ray Science and Technology. 2019;**27**(1):139–147

[33] Keshtkar M, Mosleh-Shirazi MA, Saba V. Assessment of the effectiveness of Saba shielding with the composition of Cu–Bi in neck CT imaging: A phantom and patient study. Journal of Radiological Protection. 2023;**43**(4):041503. DOI: 10.1088/1361-6498/acffd4

[34] Sikand M, Stinchcombe S, Livesley PJ. Study on the use of gonadal protection shields during paediatric pelvic X-rays. Annals of the Royal College of Surgeons of England. 2003;**85**(6):422–425. DOI: 10.1308/003588403322520852

[35] Larjava HRS, Eneh CTM, Niiniviita HM. To shield or not to shield: Shielding may have unintended effects on patient dose in CT. European Radiology. 2024;**34**(4):2480–2486

[36] Yildizer Keriş E. Effect of patient anxiety on image motion artefacts in CBCT. BMC Oral Health. 2017;**17**(1):73 DOI: 10.1186/s12903-017-0367-4

[37] Heyer CM, Thüring J, Lemburg SP, Kreddig N, Hasenbring M, Dohna M, et al. Anxiety of patients undergoing CT Imaging-An underestimated problem? Academic Radiology. 2015;**22**: 105–112

[38] Hedgire SS, Kalva SP. Chapter 9 - Catheter Angiography (Vascular). In Abbara S, Kalva SP, editors. Problem Solving in Cardiovascular Imaging. Philadelphia (PA): W.B. Saunders; 2013. p. 155–162. Available from: https://www.sciencedirect.com/science/article/pii/B9781437727685000097

[39] Gohmann RF, Mettke SM, Krieghoff C, Lücke C, Kaiser F, Seitz P, et al. Video-assisted informed consent in cardiac imaging: Influence on patient experience during CT—the randomized controlled VAICICI Trial.

European Radiology. 2026;**36**:148–162. DOI: 10.1007/s00330-025-11741-8.

[40] Siegel MJ. Pediatric CT angiography. European Radiology Supplements. 2005;**15**(4):d32–d36

[41] Kino A, Zucker EJ, Honkanen A, Kneebone J, Wang J, Chan F, et al. Ultrafast pediatric chest computed tomography: Comparison of free-breathing vs. breath-hold imaging with and without anesthesia in young children. Pediatric Radiology. 2019;**49** (3):301–307. DOI: 10.1007/s00247-018-4295-5

[42] Goo HW, Siripornpitak S, Chen SJ, Lilyasari O, Zhong YM, Latiff HA, et al. Pediatric cardiothoracic ct guideline provided by the asian society of cardiovascular imaging congenital heart disease study group: Part 2. contemporary clinical applications. Korean Journal of Radiology. 2021;**22**: 1397–1415

[43] Goldberg-Stein S, Liu B, Hahn PF, Lee SI. Body CT during pregnancy: Utilization trends, examination indications, and fetal radiation doses. American Journal of Roentgenology. 2011;**196**(1):146–151

[44] Acr-spr practice parameter for imaging pregnant or potentially pregnant patients with ionizing radiation

[45] Sadro CT, Dubinsky TJ. CT in pregnancy: Risks and benefits. Applied Radiology. 2013;**42**(10):6

[46] Mlynarski R, Sosnowski M, Mlynarska A, Tendera M. Computed tomography in patients with cardiac pacemakers: Difficulties and solutions. Heart and Vessels. 2012;**27**(3): 300–306

[47] McCollough CH, Zhang J, Primak AN, Clement WJ, Buysman JR. Effects of CT irradiation on implantable cardiac rhythm management devices. Radiology. 2007;**243**(3):766–774

[48] Kremer NI, Oterdoom DLM, van Laar PJ, Piña-Fuentes D, van Laar T, Drost G, et al. Accuracy of intraoperative computed tomography in deep brain stimulation—A prospective noninferiority study. Neuromodulation: Technology at the Neural Interface. 2019;**22**(4):472–477. Available from: https://www.sciencedirect.com/science/article/pii/S1094715921019371

[49] Ellis JA, Leung R, Winfree CJ. Spinal infusion pump-catheter leak detected by high-resolution 3D computed tomography: Technical note. Journal of Neurosurgery: Spine. 2011;**15** (5):555–557

[50] Kennedy TA, Connell N, Szczykutowicz T, Schafer S, Royalty K, Nace S, et al. Flat-panel CT for cochlear implant electrode imaging: comparison to multi-detector CT. Otology & Neurotology. 2016;**37**. Available from: https://journals.lww.com/otology-neurotology/fulltext/2016/12000/flat_panel_ct_for_cochlear_implant_electrode.30.aspx

[51] van der Molen AJ, Thomsen HS, Morcos SK. (ESUR) M of CMSC of ES of UR. Effect of iodinated contrast media on thyroid function in adults. European Radiology. 2004;**14**(5):902–907

[52] Silberstein EB, Alavi A, Balon HR, Clarke SEM, Divgi C, Gelfand MJ, et al. The SNMMI practice guideline for therapy of thyroid disease with 131I 3.0.

Journal of Nuclear Medicine. 2012;**53**:1633–1651

[53] Somashekar DK, Davenport MS, Cohan RH, Dillman JR, Ellis JH. Effect of intravenous low-osmolality iodinated contrast media on patients with myasthenia gravis. Radiology. 2013;**267**(3):727–734

Chapter 3

The Horizons of Computed Tomography

Mahnoor Hafeez and Javerya Sattar

Abstract

Computed Tomography (CT) – the Nobel Prize modality has revolutionized the healthcare industry for adequate patient management and outcomes. Thanks to Sir Godfrey Hounsfield for the wonderful invention! From a technical perspective, the modality focuses on the differential attenuation of body contents; because of its excellent spatial and contrast resolution, each and every body part can be imaged from "*head to Toe*". Compared to MRI, it has a shorter scan time and limited artifacts. It is an essential need of each hospital's radiology department, with referrals from A&E, stroke, ENT, neurology, trauma unit, medicine, surgery, gynecology, pediatrics, oncology, pulmonology, urology, and forensic medicine. CT not only has a role in diagnostics and triage of patients but is also a cornerstone in guided procedures and intervention. PET-CT is a new technological advancement in nuclear medicine. CT has opened new doors for radiologists' employment, including tele-radiology and worldwide machine equipment trading. CT has brought innovation in medical education via virtual dissection. Because of the ionizing radiation and cancer-related concerns, imaging appropriateness should be considered.

Keywords: CT, PET-CT, attenuation, Hounsfield, virtual dissection, appropriateness

1. Introduction

CT is a cross-sectional imaging modality based on X-rays, i.e., ionizing radiation. Its key role in guiding clinical decisions and saving patients' lives is worth mentioning! It has been the work horse in hospitals—a game changer in the diagnostic world since its invention in 1973! The CT scan creates a roadmap and GPS for a surgeon in operative procedures. It also helps in the assessment of post-operative, post-chemo – radiotherapy complications, as well as recurrent and residual neoplastic disease. In this chapter, insights, scope, CT hazards and concerns, practical concepts, latest advancements, and the authors' experience related to the modality are presented.

2. Physics, dosimetry, techniques and CT protocols

CT has an excellent ability to characterize the three states of matter, i.e., air, solid, and liquid, and to further sub-characterize solid tissues based upon attenuation.

IntechOpen

The human eye can appreciate 32 shades of gray subjectively. Tissues can be further characterized based upon attenuation quantitatively on an attenuation scale ranging from +3,000 to -1,000 Hounsfield units (HU) (for example: air [-300], fat [-70 to -200], fluid [0 to 20], gray matter [40], white matter [45], muscle [50], bone [1000], and metal [3000]) [1, 2]. CT can diagnose calcification, hemorrhage, wood, glass, metal, foreign body/gossypiboma based on HU values.

There has been a transition from step-and-shoot CT to helical (single slice) to MDCT 16 up to -256 slice scanners [2]. Of the four generations of CT, most of the scanners are of the 3rd-gen rotate-rotate type, thanks to slip-ring technology for simultaneous X-ray tube and detector array rotation in a gantry.

Spatial ability is the ability to separate two lines in an image to see fine details, and in CT, it is limited to 20 lines/cm, while contrast resolution is the ability to distinguish soft tissue structures regardless of shape or size. Image acquisition parameters vary according to the type of study; i.e., mAs, field of view (FOV), pitch, matrix size, and slice thickness are different for high-resolution CT versus other CT studies. The image is displayed via filtered back projection, which compensates for blurring inherent in back projection, and iterative reconstruction, which solves the noise issue [3]. Technical parameters include MPR, maximum intensity projection, and volume rendering [4]. Modern CT scanners have multiple slices, up to 256, with the shortest scan times, and images can be viewed in bone, lung, and soft tissue windows, etc. CT protocols differ based on the region of interest, such as CTPA – Pulmonary Embolism Protocol, to multi-phase CT abdominal scanning, where IV contrast is delivered in multiple phases (bi-/triphasic/adrenal nodule protocol) or when imaging is performed as a single-pass acquisition (Combi Scan/Split Bolus technique). Contrast can also be administered per oral or per rectal, depending upon the need.

CT artifacts are categorized into physics-based, patient-based, and hardware-based types depending upon their etiology, including motion, metal (streak), photon starvation, cone beam, partial volume, and detector ring artifacts [4]. Numerous solutions exist to overcome these issues. For example, a bow tie filter is used in head and body imaging to homogenize the projected fan beam and eliminate fan beam artifacts. CT dosimetry parameters include Dose Length Product (DLP) measured in mGy·cm, Effective Dose (mSv), and CTDI volume (mGy). In one quality assurance research project, the Effective Dose of a CT KUB scan on 16 and 128-slice scanners was found to be under 10 mSv,-consistent with ACR recommendations [5].

3. Neuroimaging and stroke

CT scan is the primary tool for assessing intracranial haemorrhage, ischemic stroke, and altered consciousness levels, primarily due to its speed, widespread availability, and cost-effectiveness in emergency situations [6, 7, 8].

Immediate use of CT highlights the critical “time is brain” principle, which warrants emergent reperfusion therapies for ischemic stroke, particularly intravenous (IV) thrombolysis with tissue plasminogen activator (tPA) and, more recently, mechanical thrombectomy [9, 10]. Furthermore, CT allows the monitoring of treatment and further management [6].

The most immediate and critical question in acute stroke is whether it is ischemic or hemorrhagic. Intravenous thrombolysis is contraindicated in hemorrhagic stroke due to the risk of exacerbating bleeding and causing severe harm. Non-contrast head CT (NCCT) is highly sensitive for acute blood, which appears hyper dense (bright).

This rapid exclusion of hemorrhage allows clinicians to quickly determine if thrombolytic therapy can be considered, thus preventing delays that could jeopardize patient outcomes. [11]

NCCT can be performed within minutes of a patient's arrival at the emergency department (ED). Guidelines emphasize minimizing the "door-to-CT" time, typically targeting 20–25 minutes from ED arrival to CT scan initiation [12].

Early ischemic signs on NCCT are hyper dense artery sign, decreased gray-white matter differentiation, cytotoxic edema (due to breakdown of the blood-brain barrier, manifested as hypodensity) (**Figure 1**), and mass effect [13].

Alberta Stroke Program Early CT Score (ASPECTS) is a quantitative imaging tool with a 10-point validated grading system designed to quantify ischemic changes in the middle cerebral artery (MCA) territory on NCCT. The 10 zones include the caudate nucleus, lentiform nucleus, internal capsule, insular cortex, and six MCA territory cortices: the initial three at, and the later three above the level of the basal ganglia. It has been employed as a surrogate marker for infarct size, with a score of 7 commonly used as the threshold for thrombolysis [14]. A low ASPECTS score suggests a larger ischemic core and is unlikely to achieve a good outcome [14].

Vascular imaging, including CT angiography (CTA) and CT perfusion (CTP), is considered for further assessment in stroke patients. CTA allows detailed visualization of the cerebrovascular anatomy and pathology (**Figure 2**) i.e., large vessel occlusion, direct visualization of the thrombus, localization of the site of the occlusion, and collateral circulation [6], and aids in possible endovascular intervention in patients with acute ischemic stroke.

CT perfusion is a dynamic imaging technique that measures brain hemodynamics and provides quantitative maps of cerebral blood flow (CBF), cerebral blood volume (CBV), and mean transit time (MTT) or time to peak (TTP). Therefore, CTP allows the physiological assessment for the derivation of the ischemic core (irreversibly damaged tissue) and the ischemic penumbra (hypo-perfused, ischemic but

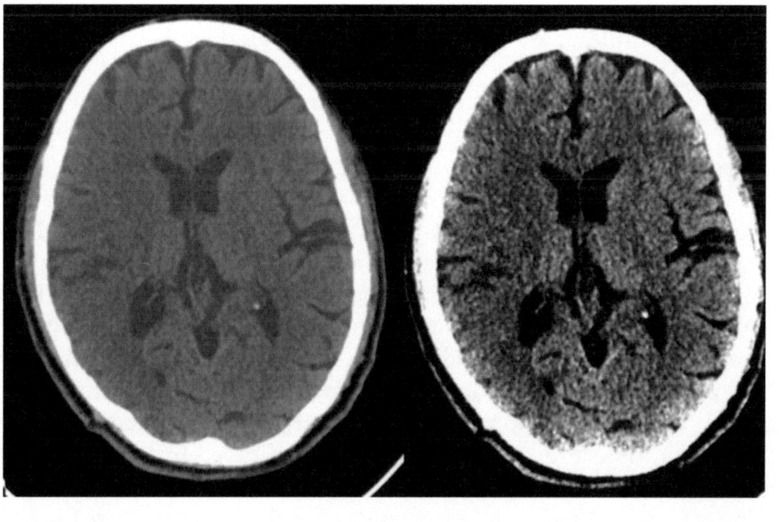

Figure 1.
CT brain axial section (soft tissue window-Left and stroke window-Rgiht): Right middle cerebral artery ischemic infarct is depicted by hypo attenuation and loss of the gray-white matter differentiation (cerebral edema) in the right fronto-temporal region.

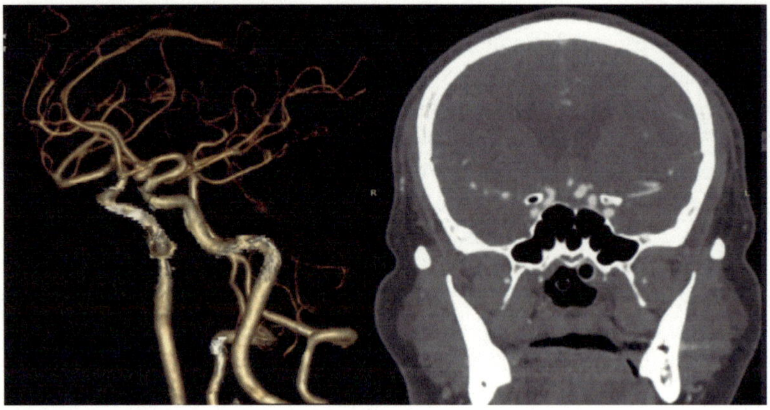

Figure 2.
Saccular aneurysm of the A1 segment of the left anterior cerebral artery.

salvageable tissue) and facilitates the calculation of the mismatch volume. CTP identifies the tissue at risk that can be salvaged, i.e., the ischemic penumbra.

Nevertheless, a radiologist must recognize stroke mimics to avoid misdiagnosis. The most common stroke mimics on CT imaging are seizure (postictal state presented as focal cortical swelling/subtle hypodensity), hypoglycemic state (diffuse low-density in the cortex or basal ganglia), space-occupying lesion (heterogeneous density with mass effect, with or without calcification), encephalitis (mostly hypodensities in the temporal lobes), subdural hematoma, and toxic or metabolic encephalopathy (diffuse cerebral edema with loss of gray-white matter differentiation). If CT appears inconclusive, an MRI of the brain is necessary.

4. Petrous temporal bone

It is the most complex part of human anatomy. High-resolution CT (HRCT) of the petrous temporal bone is the investigation of choice. External ear anomalies include microtia, meatal atresia, atretic plate, and usually co-exist with Temporomandibular joint dysfunction and middle ear anomalies (hypoplastic ossicles) [15]. Syndromes associated with it are hemifacial microsomia, Treacher-Collins syndrome (branchial apparatus anomaly), and Goldenhar-Gorlin syndrome (facio-auriculo-vertebral dysplasia). Congenital vascular masses include aberrant ICA and high-riding jugular bulb. Inner ear anomalies include Michel anomaly (total aplasia), Mondini anomaly, otocyst, and absent semicircular canals. HRCT is also recommended for the pre-operative assessment of cochlear implant insertion. Absence of the basal turn of the cochlea precludes surgery for cochlear implant.

Acquired pathologies include acute otitis media (OM), which can lead to tympanic membrane perforation, chronic suppurative otitis media (CSOM), and coalescent mastoiditis – a radiological diagnosis indicated by cell wall breakdown (muco-periosteal inflammation). Its further complications include Bezold's abscess (sternocleidomastoid), Citelli's abscess (posterior digastric triangle) via erosion of the medial mastoid cortex, internal jugular vein (IJV) thrombosis, skull base osteomyelitis, petrous apicitis, and Gradenigo syndrome. CSOM has two types: tubo-tympanic (safe) and attico-antral (dangerous), which can lead to ossicular

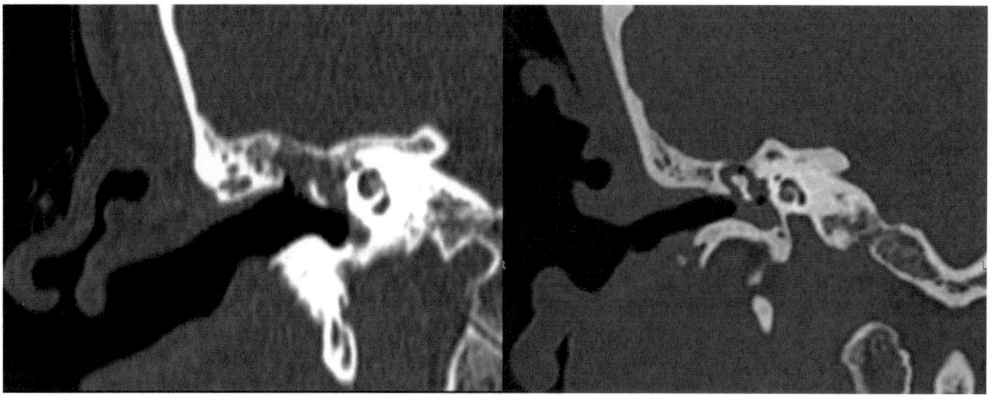

Figure 3.
Sagittal HRCT temporal bone shows cholesteatoma with scutum and ossicular erosion (left) and CSOM (left).

disruption and facial nerve dehiscence, cerebrospinal fluid (CSF) fistula (lateral semi-circular canal erosion), cholesteatoma, labyrinthitis, intracranial abscess, and dural venous sinus thrombosis.

Cholesteatoma (keratinized stratified squamous epithelial mass) can be divided into pars flaccida/pars tensa type and congenital/acquired etiology. It can be differentiated from CSOM via mass effect (expansion of aditus), anti-dependent (attic) location, and lack of fluid level (**Figure 3**). Malignant otitis externa can be difficult to differentiate from squamous cell carcinoma of the external auditory canal, as both present with a discharging ear, nerve palsies, and have the same radiologic presentation [16]. Histopathology is the gold standard in such cases.

Glomus tumor presents as a pulsatile vascular mass visible through the tympanic membrane and can be classified as Glomus tympanicum or jugulo-tympanicum with intracranial or cervical extension. For its evaluation and to determine its extent, contrast-enhanced CT or MRI is necessary. Trauma can be divided into longitudinal or transverse fractures in relation to the axis of the petrous temporal bone. Important facts to report include ossicular dislocation, facial canal dehiscence, and mastoid or tegmen tympani fractures.

5. CT paranasal sinuses, face and musculoskeletal system

As per ACR appropriateness criteria, CT PNS is recommended for the evaluation of acute complicated sinusitis, chronic rhino-sinusitis, and to diagnose intra-cranial and intra-orbital complications. It is useful for diagnosing fungal sinusitis because of its metallic contents. It is also useful for diagnosing PNS variants (e.g., Haller cells, agger nasi, optic nerve variants), pre and post-FESS assessment, and suspected CSF leak [17, 18]. Chronic rhino-sinusitis has five distinct patterns, i.e., infundibular pattern – (obstruction of the maxillary infundibulum resulting in isolated maxillary sinusitis), osteomeatal unit pattern – (middle meatal obstruction results in maxillary, anterior ethmoid, and frontal sinusitis), spheno-ethmoid recess pattern – (obstruction results in posterior ethmoid and sphenoid sinusitis), sino-nasal polyposis pattern (sino-nasal polyps, with opacification of various sinuses), and sporadic/unclassifiable pattern, which includes retention cysts and mucoceles [19].

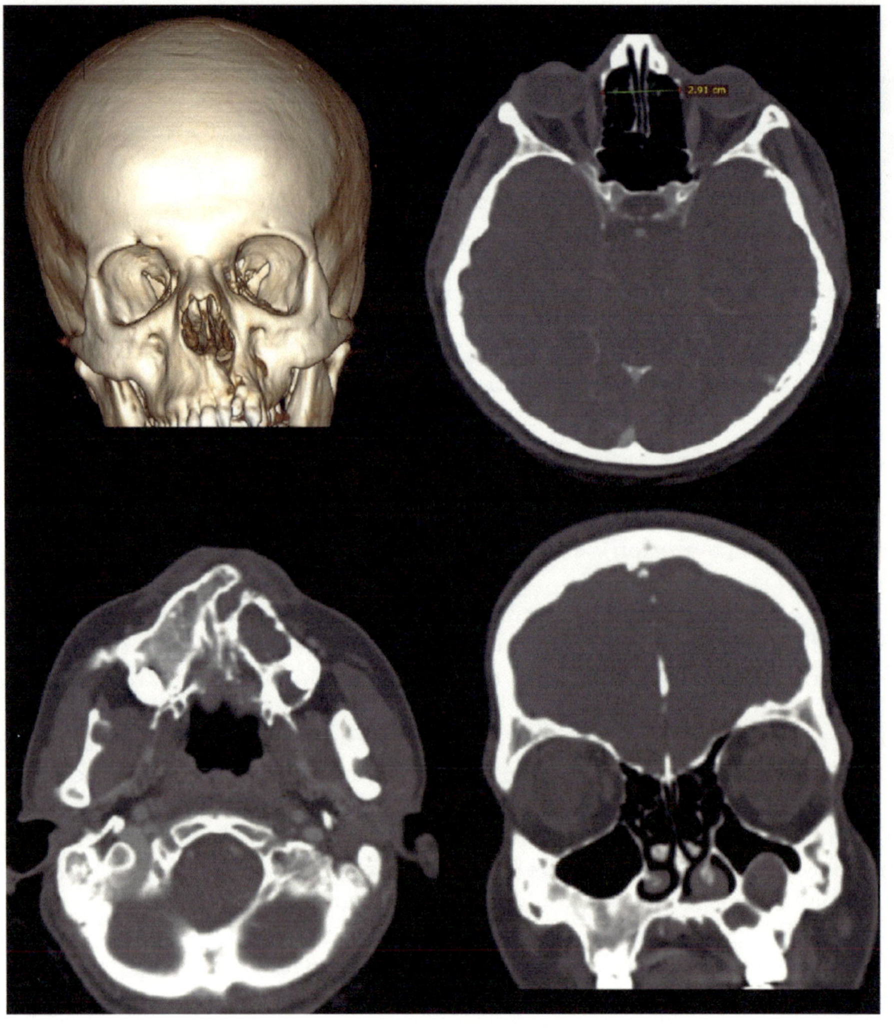

Figure 4.
CT face of a 25 years old female with Gorlin-Goltz, i.e., Left sided cleft palate, odontogenic keratocysts, hypertelorism with increased inter orbital, and dural calcification.

CT scan of the face with 3D reformatting is used to evaluate craniofacial anomalies, including cleft lip and palate (**Figure 4**), and hemifacial microsomia; its types and severity are assessed according to the OMENS (orbit, mandible, ear, nerve, soft tissues) classification [20, 21, 22].

CT scan is also indicated for post-operative spine assessment for the positioning of prosthesis and the etiology of scoliosis, e.g., vertebral segmentation anomalies. It is also useful to assess cartilaginous tumors and osteoid osteoma.

6. CT in cardiovascular imaging

Although cardiac MRI is the gold standard modality for cardiac anomalies, ECG-gated cardiac CT is indicated for the evaluation of cardiovascular anomalies and cardiac masses. CT Coronary Angiography indicates vessel stenosis

DOI: http://dx.doi.org/10.5772/intechopen.1013395

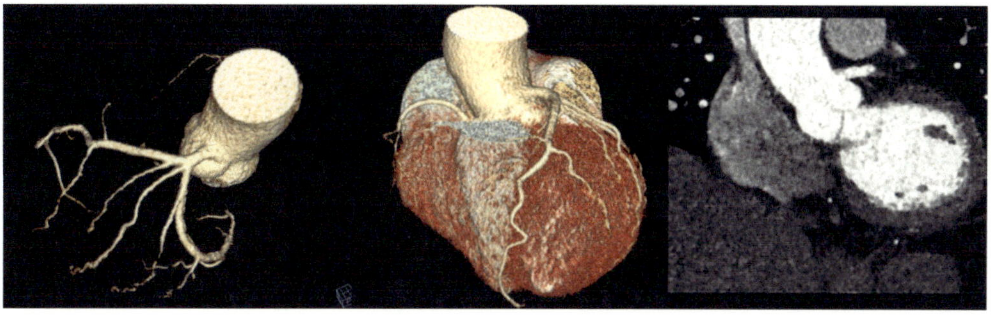

Figure 5.
CT coronary angiography of a 55 years old female with MIP, volume-rendered and source images.

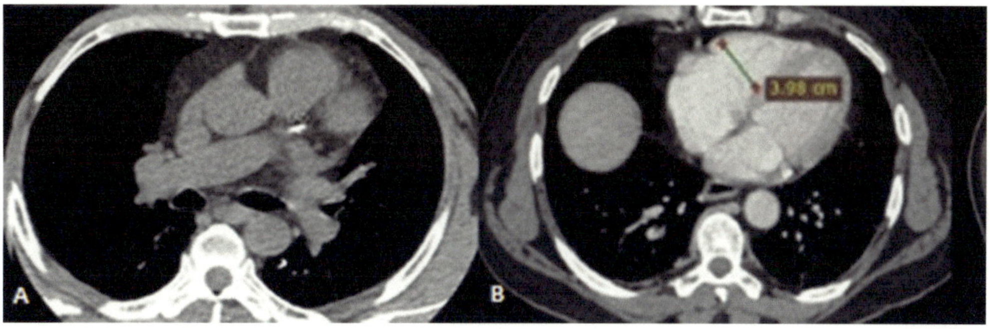

Figure 6.
(a) A 48-year-old male with a coronary calcium score of 78 shows left LAD calcification. (b) NEGCT with cardiac chamber size assessment.

(hemodynamically significant vs. insignificant; mild, moderate, or severe), and post-CABG is useful for assessing vessel patency (**Figure 5**). NICE has recommended it as 1st line test for chronic stable chest pain of suspected cardiac origin. Its advanced uses include cardiac fractional flow reserve (FFR), trans-catheter aortic valve implantation (TAVI) measurements, and delayed CT left atrial appendage thrombus exclusion for ablation in atrial fibrillation (100% NPV) [23, 24].

It has a few advantages over cardiac MRI, i.e., it is quick and safe, and it has no MR safety issues (pacemakers, drip stands, and oxygen cylinders). MRI is limited by artifacts, including cardiac motion, breath-hold, motion blooming artifacts, etc. On the other hand, Non ECG-gated cardiac CT (NEGCT) can assess cardiac chamber sizes accurately (**Figure 6**) as well as aortic diseases, e.g., aneurysm and dissection. Plain CT chest can raise suspicion of anemia via chambers' blood attenuation measurements [25–30].

7. CT angiography (CTA) and transplant imaging

CTA is considered a workhorse for diagnosing vascular emergencies. It can evaluate active bleeds and arterial disruption, either thrombus or occlusion, dissections, dural arteriovenous fistula, aneurysm, pseudo aneurysm, graft tear/infections [31]. CT pulmonary angiography evaluates pulmonary thromboembolism/infarct.

CT remains the cornerstone of transplant medicine. It plays an integral role in both pre-transplant donor and post-transplant recipient assessment for complications across a range of solid organ transplants, including liver, kidney, lung, and heart [32]. It delineates the donor's and recipient's anatomical structures and provides detailed 3D visualization of vascular anatomy, enabling precise pre-surgical planning for organ donation. In liver transplantation, CT angiography evaluates hepatic vasculature, liver volume, and quantifies hepatic fat content, contributing to donor selection and risk assessment. Additionally, CT aids in oncological staging, such as hepatocellular carcinoma (HCC), to determine transplant eligibility. In renal transplantation, it evaluates renal vessels and identifies accessory arteries. In lung transplantation, it identifies airway anastomotic patency.

CT is indispensable for the early detection of postoperative complications, including hemorrhage, infection, abscess formation, vascular thrombosis, lymphoceles, and graft rejection. It can identify the recurrence of primary diseases and the development of post-transplant malignancies [33].

8. Whole body CT imaging [WBCT]

It refers to the cross-sectional imaging of the head, neck, chest, abdomen, and pelvis. Section-wise imaging is recommended for infective/inflammatory and neoplastic etiology. Whole-body CT scan [WB CT] is useful for polytrauma patients. In addition to head and neck malignancies, CT helps in differentiating cervical reactive vs. metastatic lymphadenopathy [34].

There are clear-cut indications for when to recommend contrast-enhanced CT (CECT) chest versus HRCT chest for respiratory pathologies. Clinicians do sometimes confuse "what to request when". CECT chest is used for the evaluation of hemoptysis, staging, pleuro-pulmonary and mediastinal masses, abscesses, pneumonia, thoracic empyema, its etiology, trauma, post-operative cases, and transplant pulmonary complications, while HRCT chest is utilized for the assessment of tuberculosis parenchymal involvement, interstitial lung disease, pneumoconiosis, viral infections (e.g., COVID), airway diseases, and ABPA (**Figure 7**) [35]. Plain chest CT is ideal for differentiating giant bullae from pneumothorax, as the

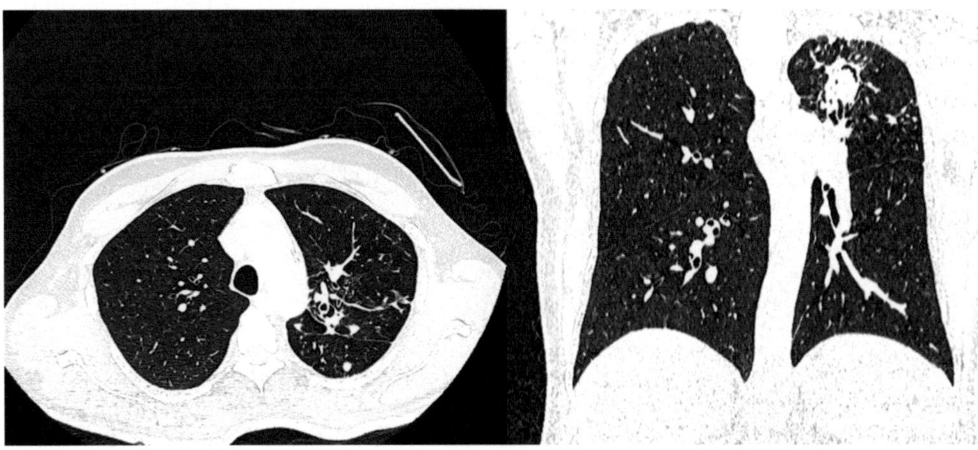

Figure 7.
Active pulmonary tuberculosis: a patient referred from Ojha Institute of Chest Diseases who underwent HRCT chest shows tree-in-bud, centrilobular nodules in upper lobar distribution—implies granulomatous infection with mycetoma.

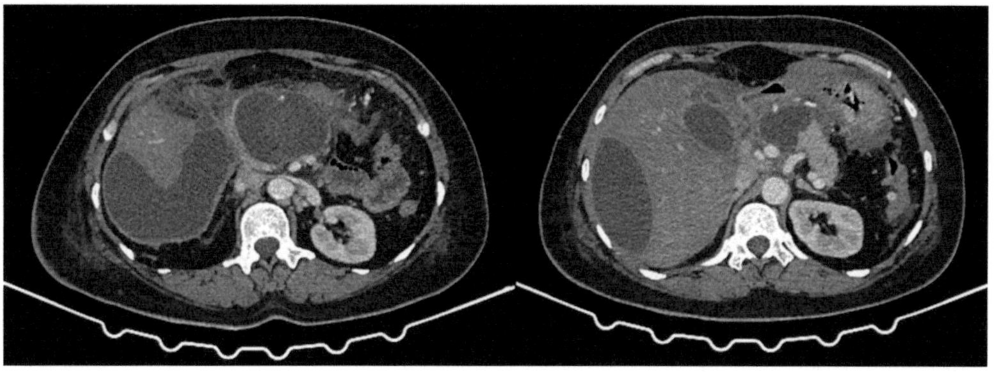

Figure 8.
43 – year-old male with acute pancreatitis, pancreatic walled-off necrosis, sub-hepatic collections.

management approaches for the two are different—the former requires bullectomy, and the latter requires chest tube insertion [36].

It has a role in the evaluation of acute pancreatitis (**Figure 8**), complicated cholecystitis, enterocolitis, peritonitis, biliary masses and strictures, hepatic abscesses, splenic infarction/abscess, appendicitis, diverticulitis, inflammatory bowel diseases, bowel wall ischemia, and gastrointestinal perforation. CECT helps to differentiate types of acute pancreatitis: interstitial edematous or necrotizing, and its complications like pancreatic pseudocyst. The CT scoring system provides prognostic information. CT can diagnose the transition point in bowel obstruction and its underlying cause.

Thin-section CECT has high accuracy for choledocholithiasis and should be utilized for obstructive jaundice when MRCP is not available [37, 38]. Despite the widespread use of ultrasound in assessing gynecological disorders, CT is also used to assess ovarian torsion, ovarian cysts, and pelvic inflammatory disease. A CT scan is also useful for evaluating pelvic inflammatory disease, its complications, obstetric emergencies, C-section complications, as well as pathways of extra-pelvic spread of pelvic disease [39, 40].

9. Role of CT in emergencies

9.1 Traumatic emergencies

CT is the preferred imaging modality for evaluating acute trauma in the emergency department due to its speed and accessibility [41, 42]. Due to its widespread availability, speed, and ability to diagnose subtle as well as significant injuries, a CT scan is preferably installed in the trauma bay to limit transportation and diagnostic time [42].

There are two main strategies for CT scanning in the emergency department. The first one is Whole-Body CT (WBCT) for severely injured patients, and the other is focused CT protocols for stable patients with a specific, localized injury.

Whole-body CT (WBCT) is a comprehensive diagnostic imaging modality used for hemodynamically unstable patients with major trauma to identify critical multisystem injuries expeditiously. This protocol typically involves an initial non-contrast acquisition of the head and cervical spine, followed by a single-pass, contrast-enhanced scan of the chest, abdomen, and pelvis. To refine diagnostics, variations may be employed, such as split-bolus or delayed imaging techniques, which are optimized for specific evaluations, such as assessing urinary tract trauma or active hemorrhage [43, 44].

Biphasic CT is a contrast injection technique that captures images during two distinct phases – the arterial and portal venous – to obtain detailed information about both the blood supply and organ parenchymal injuries. In some trauma centers, a WBCT protocol may incorporate a biphasic or modified biphasic technique for the contrast-enhanced portion of the scan, often for the chest, abdomen, and pelvis [45].

A common variation used in trauma is a split-bolus, single-pass protocol, which can be described as a modified biphasic approach. This is done to reduce total radiation dose and imaging time while still providing detailed information for detecting a wide range of injuries. This protocol is typically performed after a preliminary non-contrast CT study of the abdomen and pelvis to rule out kidney stones. The procedure involves administering two separate intravenous injections of contrast medium (50 mL each dose) – the first bolus initiates nephrographic enhancement, and the second, administered after a precise delay (of 8 minutes), enables simultaneous visualization of the excretory phase. The single acquisition following the second injection effectively captures these combined phases, optimizing diagnostic information while prioritizing dose reduction [46, 47].

Focused CT protocols involve targeted scans for stable trauma patients to minimize radiation exposure, with specific imaging techniques that include non-contrast scans for the head and cervical spine, angiograms (CTA) for assessing major chest vessels, contrast-enhanced scans for abdominal and pelvic injuries, performing CT cystography for suspected bladder injury to differentiate intra- or extra-peritoneal bladder rupture, and specialized pediatric protocols adjusted for children's radiation sensitivity.

MDCT using a dual-phase scanning protocol in poly trauma is the diagnostic modality of choice. [48] CT examination not only assists in the accurate detection of traumatic injuries but also categorizes patients as suitable for either radiological intervention management (via angio-embolization) or surgical management, thus being paramount in-timely bleeding control and reducing morbidity. [49]

In patients with cranio-cerebral injuries, a CT scan is performed to evaluate fractures, extra-axial hemorrhage including subdural, epidural (**Figure 9**), intra-ventricular or subarachnoid hemorrhage, intra parenchymal contusions or hematomas, or diffuse axonal shearing, but it can also diagnose secondary impacts such as contre-coup injury, cerebral edema, and herniation. Follow-up imaging is often required in patients to monitor rebleeding or assess post-intervention complications [50].

For the evaluation of thoraco-abdominal pelvic trauma, CT detects free intra-abdominal fluid and pneumothorax, thus selecting hemo-dynamically unstable patients presenting with severe hemo-peritoneum or pneumothorax for immediate intervention. MDCT has surpassed e-FAST ultrasound for the detection of visceral injuries [51].

The American Association for the Surgery of Trauma (AAST) has developed a CECT injury grading scale for abdominal parenchymal solid visceral injuries in order to guide management. The spleen is the most commonly affected abdominal organ. Most blunt liver and splenic injuries are managed non-surgically. The AAST

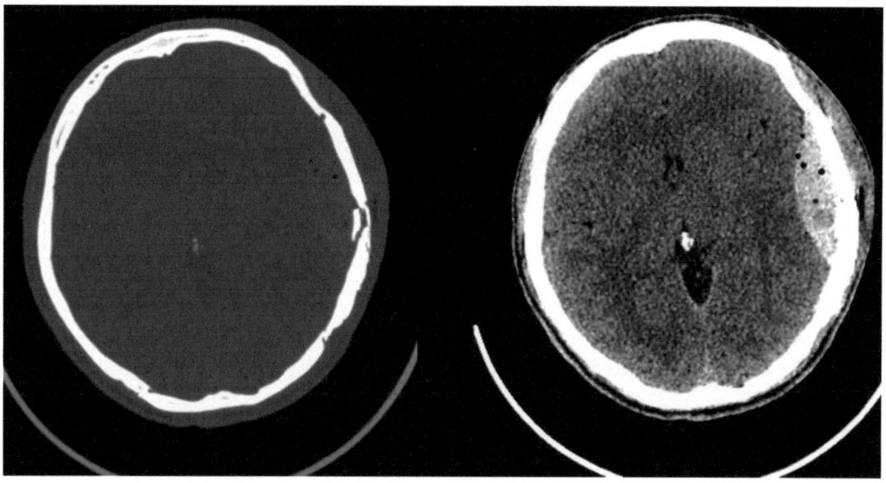

Figure 9.
Left temporal bone fractures and left-sided epidural hematoma with swirl sign representing active arterial extravasation.

injury criteria grade the severity of injury according to the size and location of lacerations and hematomas. Higher-grade injuries (those graded 3 and above) usually require surgical management. In short, dedicated clinical assessment and hemodynamic status, along with CT findings, determine the management plan: conservative management, angioembolization via interventional radiology, or surgery. CT scans detect traumatic injuries, including contusions, lacerations, hematomas, renal injury, urinary leaks, pancreatic parenchymal/ductal injuries, and bowel perforation [42]. On CT scans, active hemorrhage appears as a contrast blush sign in the viscera, which persists or grows larger on delayed imaging, in contrast to a pseudo-aneurysm or AV fistula, where contrast washes out on delayed-phase images.

Hollow viscus and mesenteric injuries with blunt abdominal trauma can be subtle, but their identification is crucial in order to reduce morbidity and mortality secondary to peritonitis and sepsis. Transection or focal discontinuity in the bowel wall, pneumo-peritoneum, and adjacent free peritoneal fluid are considered the most specific signs of bowel injury. Other, less specific signs include abnormal bowel wall enhancement, focal wall thickening, and mesenteric fat stranding. Active extravasation from a mesenteric vessel is the most specific sign of mesenteric injury, mesenteric hematoma, or abrupt cutoff/beading of any mesenteric vessel.

Hypoperfusion complex (a combination of hyper enhancement of the bowel and diffuse wall thickening) is seen in both direct bowel injury as well as in trauma patients with persistent hypovolemia despite IV fluid resuscitation [52].

CT scan helps in assessing the hemo peritoneum [fluid with Hounsfield attenuation values ranging between 20–45 HU] as well as localizing the source of hemorrhage using the sentinel clot sign [high attenuation density fluid at the site of bleeding]. [52]

Pediatric non-accidental trauma (NAT) is a major cause of morbidity and mortality, and the prompt identification of NAT in children has a significant impact on its management and prognosis. The European Society of Pediatric Radiology has recommended imaging guidelines for suspected child abuse/NAT for children of different ages. A full skeletal survey is recommended in an infant to assess skeletal injuries. For a child older than 1 year of age, if there are any abnormal neurologic findings or any abnormal findings on the skeletal survey, then they should undergo non-contrast CT brain with 3D reformats, with further MR imaging of the brain and whole spine performed if required [53]. NCCT is a frontline imaging modality in abusive head trauma (AAT) for the identification and evaluation of subdural hematomas, skull fractures, contusions, hypoxic-ischemic parenchymal injuries, and edema [54].

9.2 Non-traumatic emergencies

CT is also recommended for the evaluation of mal-positioned chest tubes (MCT) and PEG tube complications. CT is especially useful when chest X-rays fail to adequately visualize mediastinal or pleuro-parenchymal abnormalities and can accurately assess chest tube positioning. The CT scan has better accuracy than plain chest radiograph (CXR) to evaluate MCT [55].

CXR, along with computed tomography (CT), has been the workhorse of imaging for lung parenchymal assessment in patients with COVID-19 pneumonia [56].

Fat stranding on a CT scan is considered a radiological sign in assessing the presence of inflammation within the thoraco-abdominal pelvic cavity. Abdominal fat stranding may cause hazy or ground glass-like attenuation and increased fat attenuation in severe cases [57]. It may be associated with various benign and malignant conditions. However, its presence can help direct the clinician's attention to areas of potential concern and guide further diagnostic evaluation. The fat stranding location on a CT scan can offer valuable diagnostic clues. Acute cholecystitis may be suggested in the right upper quadrant; acute pancreatitis or pyelonephritis may be suggested in the left upper quadrant. Fat stranding in the right lower quadrant often indicates appendicitis, omental infarction, or Crohn's disease, whereas in the left lower quadrant, it commonly points to diverticulitis or bowel ischemia. Central abdominal fat stranding has a broader differential, including infectious enteritis or colitis, inflammatory bowel disease, mesenteric panniculitis, postoperative changes, and, more rarely, colon cancer [55].

10. Oncology

The widespread application of CT spans the entire continuum of cancer care – including early detection, precise staging, treatment planning, and post-therapy monitoring – establishing it as an essential tool in contemporary oncological practice [58]. Preoperative MDCT imaging plays a crucial role in patient selection and surgical planning.

Chest and abdominal CECT are indispensable in assessing tumor burden, mediastinal nodal involvement, evaluating tumor extent, and detecting regional lymphadenopathy and distant metastases for diagnosis and staging. The American Joint Committee on Cancer (AJCC) TNM system is widely used for staging, incorporating tumor invasion depth (T), nodal involvement (N), and metastasis (M) to stratify prognosis and guide treatment [59].

CT in head and neck malignancies with the puffed cheek technique (**Figure 10**) excels in assessing tumor extent, bone invasion, lymphadenopathy, and airways,

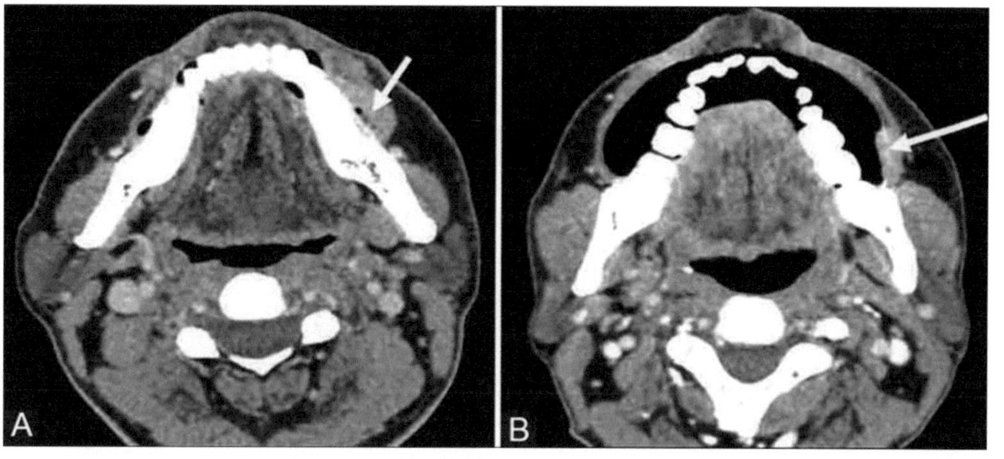

Figure 10.
(a) Contrast axial CT head at the level of the mandible showing an enhancing soft tissue density seen in the left buccal region, which is better depicted in, arising from the buccal mucosa via the puffed cheek technique.

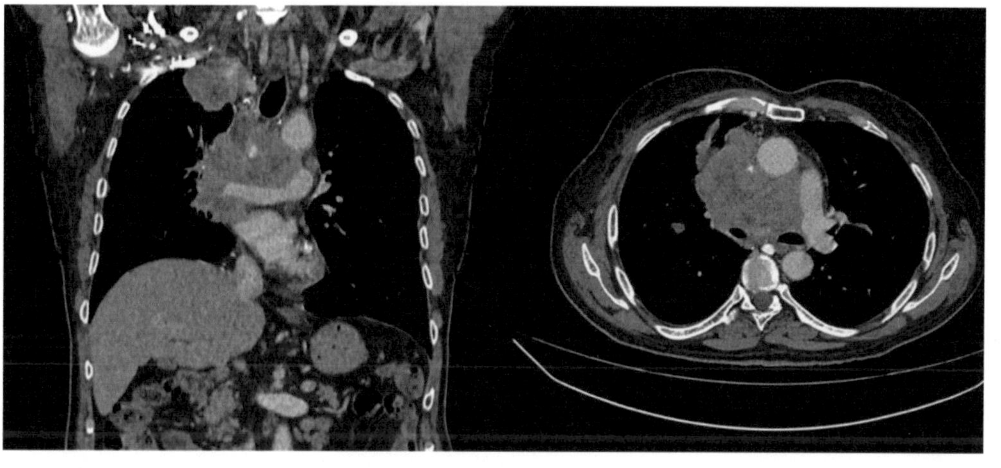

Figure 11.
Pancoast tumor (right apical mass) with pulmonary metastasis and mediastinal lymphadenopathy with superior vena cava invasion.

making it particularly useful in oral cavity, oropharynx, and larynx cancers. It is superior to MRI for evaluating cortical bone destruction [60, 61].

The IASLC (International Association for the Study of Lung Cancer) TNM staging system is the standard for categorizing tumors by size, location, nodal spread, and presence of metastases (**Figure 11**).[62]

Response Evaluation Criteria for Solid Tumors (RECIST) – a standard objective criterion to measure the response of a tumor to treatment. Similarly, Choi criteria are indicated for tumor response assessment of gastrointestinal stromal tumors (GIST).

PET CT is a modern hybrid modality that fuses computed tomography and positron emission tomography for simultaneous data presentation, i.e., anatomical–functional imaging. It involves radiopharmaceutical administration and is used primarily in the staging and treatment response of cancers (**Figure 12**) [63].

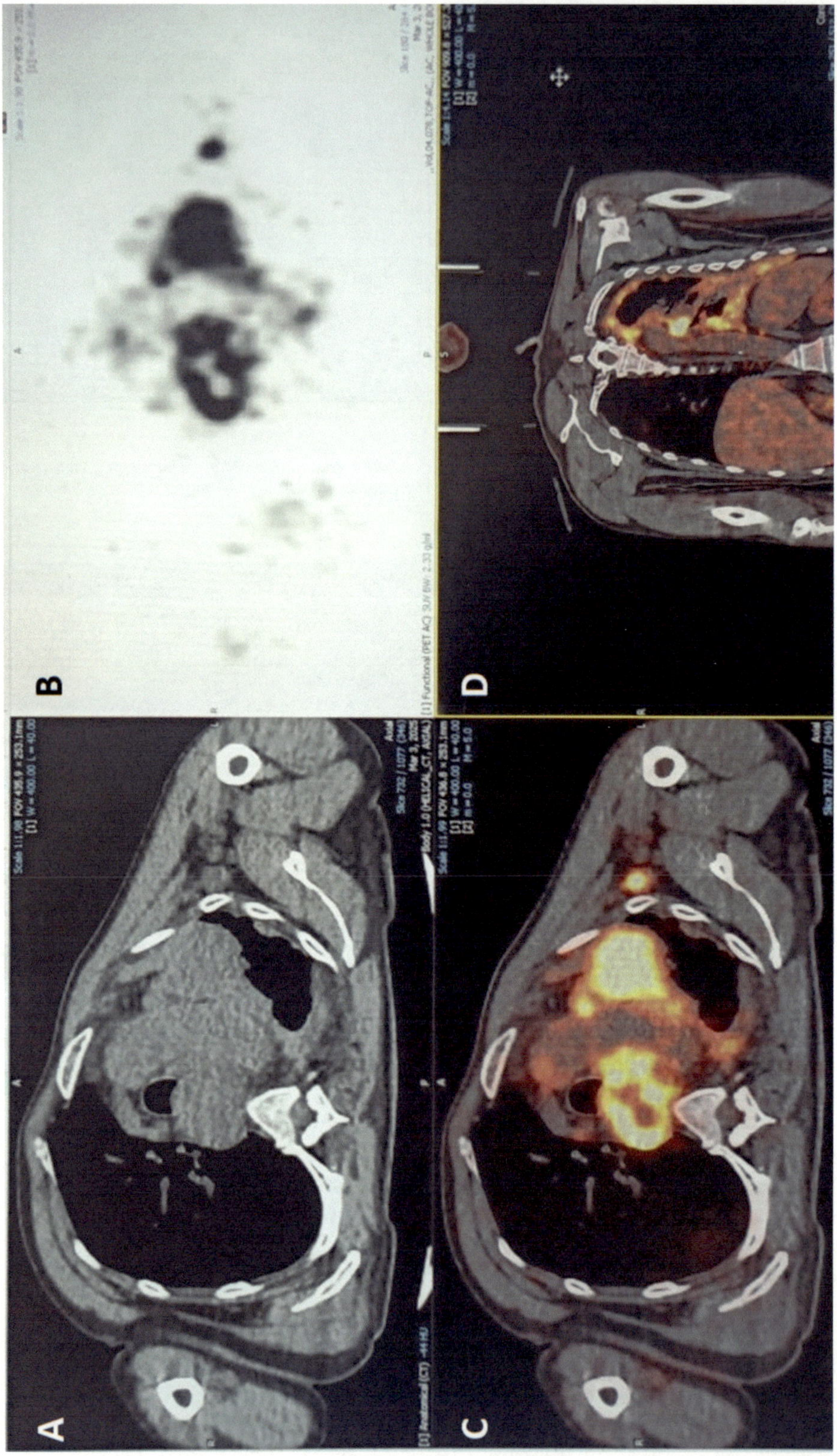

Figure 12.
61 years old male, CT only (a), PET only (b), Multi-planar PET-CT hybrid (c, d) . Known case of malignant mesothelioma with status post-chemotherapy, nodular masses along the mediastinal pleura with high SUV value and mediastinal lymph nodal deposit. Image courtesy: Dr. Nida Ihsan, Department of Radiology at Jinnah Postgraduate Medical center (JPMC).

For the staging of esophageal cancer, PET/CT or contrast-enhanced CT of the chest and abdomen is typically appropriate to assess distant nodal and metastatic disease, which is pivotal in guiding treatment decisions. The identification of metastatic spread at this stage often shifts the therapeutic approach from surgical intervention to palliative care. During treatment, particularly neo adjuvant chemotherapy, PET/CT is useful not only for evaluating the tumor's response but also for detecting any emerging new metastases. Following the completion of therapy, PET/CT or CT imaging remains appropriate for assessing potential recurrence or metastatic progression, regardless of whether a clinical suspicion of recurrence exists [33].

Ann Arbor classification is the staging system for lymphoma. CT scans, often integrated with PET, are used to assess nodal and extra-nodal involvement. PET/CT offers greater sensitivity and specificity and can upstage lymphoma in up to 40% of cases, while CT remains valuable, especially when PET findings are equivocal or non-FDG-avid [64].

CT, particularly using a pancreatic protocol with arterial and portal venous phases, is the modality of choice for staging pancreatic adenocarcinoma. It assesses tumor size, vascular encasement (key for determining resectability), and distant metastases [65]. CT accurately detects pancreatic neuroendocrine tumors (PNETs) and hyper-vascular liver metastases during multiphase scanning [66].

In colorectal cancer, CT of the chest, abdomen, and pelvis is used to detect distant metastases and to guide neo-adjuvant therapy. A meta-analysis concluded that helical CT demonstrates high sensitivity for identifying colorectal liver metastases [67, 68].

For renal cell carcinoma, MDCT has high accuracy in detecting renal vein and inferior vena cava tumor thrombus (negative predictive value ~97%, positive predictive value ~92%), facilitating preoperative strategy [69].

For ovarian malignancies, the European Society of Urogenital Radiology (ESUR) guidelines recommend contrast-enhanced CT scans covering the thorax, abdomen, and pelvis, with structured reporting to detect disease extent and assist in surgical planning, particularly to identify lesions impacting cyto-reduction feasibility. Gynecological malignancies, i.e., uterine, ovarian, and cervical cancers, are evaluated by the International Federation of Gynecology and Obstetrics (FIGO) system. [70] For cervical cancers, while PET/CT is preferred for nodal staging,

CT urography is critical in urothelial cancers for local staging and upper tract involvement detection. It shows high specificity (91–95%) but moderate sensitivity (30–53%) for nodal metastases. The AJCC TNM system classifies bladder cancer based on the depth of invasion into bladder wall layers, which is assessed on MRI; however, CT aids in the detection of nodal spread and metastasis, thus guiding prognosis and treatment [71].

CT tri-phasic study has a role in Pre and post-trans-arterial Chemo-Embolization (TACE) assessment of hepatoma. Regarding bone tumors, chondrosarcoma is better assessed on CT because of its calcified chondroid matrix.

Peritoneal carcinomatosis (PC) originates from peritoneal malignancies and may be managed through complete cyto-reductive surgery (CRS). Surgical eligibility is determined using the Peritoneal Cancer Index (PCI), with a score of ≥20 typically indicating unresectable disease. Correlating imaging findings with intraoperative observations facilitates effective teamwork between a radiologist and surgeon. CT PCI is calculated based on CT findings (size and number of peritoneal deposits in 13 locations of the abdomen) and plays an important role in multidisciplinary discussions, although its correlation with surgical PCI remains variable (**Figure 13**) [72, 73].

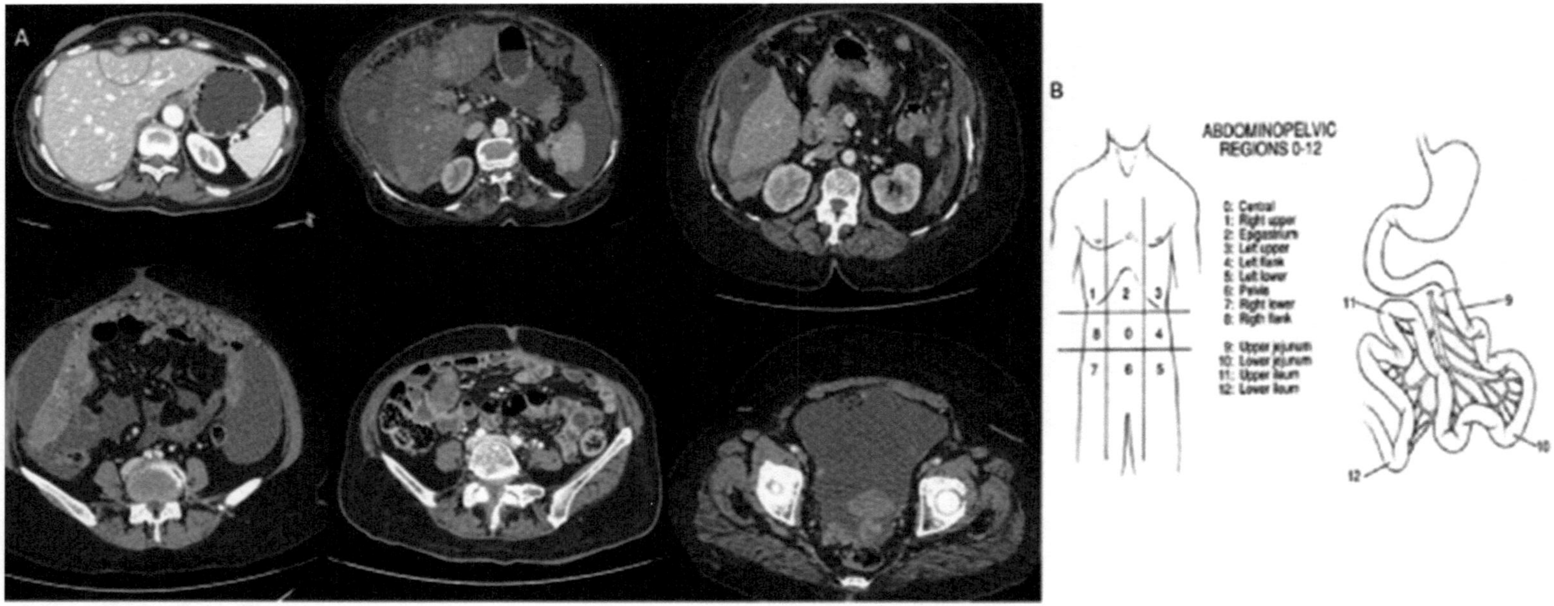

Figure 13.
Axial contrast CT sections of the abdomen show subcapsular, intrahepatic fissure, Morrison's pouch, omental, mesenteric, and deposits. B: Measurement method of peritoneal carcinomatosis index estimation.

11. Urology

CT KUB is the investigation of choice for acute flank pain. It accurately assesses stone size, density, location, and level of obstruction (**Figure 12**). Because of the soft tissue blooming artifact that exaggerates the size of the stone, the bone window is ideal for measuring stone size. These stone parameters help the urologist in choosing management options for the patient, whether the patient should undergo extracorporeal shock wave lithotripsy (ESWL), ureteroscopy and stone retrieval, conservative management, or pyelonephrolithotomy (PCNL) (**Figure 14**). CT Urogram is recommended for the evaluation of urinary tract masses, strictures, and ureteral injury. CT cystogram is useful for identifying bladder rupture or post-operative bladder injury [74–81].

The split-bolus technique, a sophisticated CT imaging protocol, is not only used in post-trauma patients but also for evaluating hematuria, as it acquires both the nephrographic (renal enhancement) and excretory (urinary tract) phases in a single scan.

12. Forensic medicine

Virtual autopsy, also known as *virtopsy*, is a non-invasive postmortem examination technique that utilizes advanced imaging modalities such as computed tomography (CT), magnetic resonance imaging (MRI), and 3D surface scanning to assess the cause of death. Unlike conventional autopsies that require dissection, virtual autopsies preserve the integrity of the body, making them particularly valuable in cases where religious, cultural, or legal constraints limit invasive procedures. This method enables high-resolution visualization of skeletal structures, internal organs, and traumatic injuries, and can be complemented by postmortem angiography or CT-guided biopsies for enhanced diagnostic accuracy. While it offers advantages such as rapid digital documentation, remote consultation, and superior detection of certain findings (e.g., gas embolism, vertebral fractures), it may have limitations in identifying some microscopic and soft tissue pathologies. Virtual autopsy has gained increasing application in forensic investigations, natural death evaluations, pediatric cases, and mass disaster scenarios [82].

Postmortem CT (PMCT) is as effective as a traditional autopsy in detecting pulmonary infections and determining natural causes of death. Additionally, it is superior in identifying vertebral fractures, which can help rule out hanging and support evidence of spinal trauma [83].

13. CT guided intervention, virtual dissection, AI, and other advancements

CT-guided interventional radiology uses percutaneous, minimally invasive techniques to perform diagnostic and therapeutic medical procedures, including biopsy, fluid aspiration, drainage, and ablation [84].

CT has brought innovation in medical education, i.e., Virtual Dissection (**Figure 15**). It is a technique in which a virtual human body can be cut into thin sections noninvasively. The usage of Computed Tomography in 2D and 3D forms is a cost-effective technique that employs high-level IT development [85, 86].

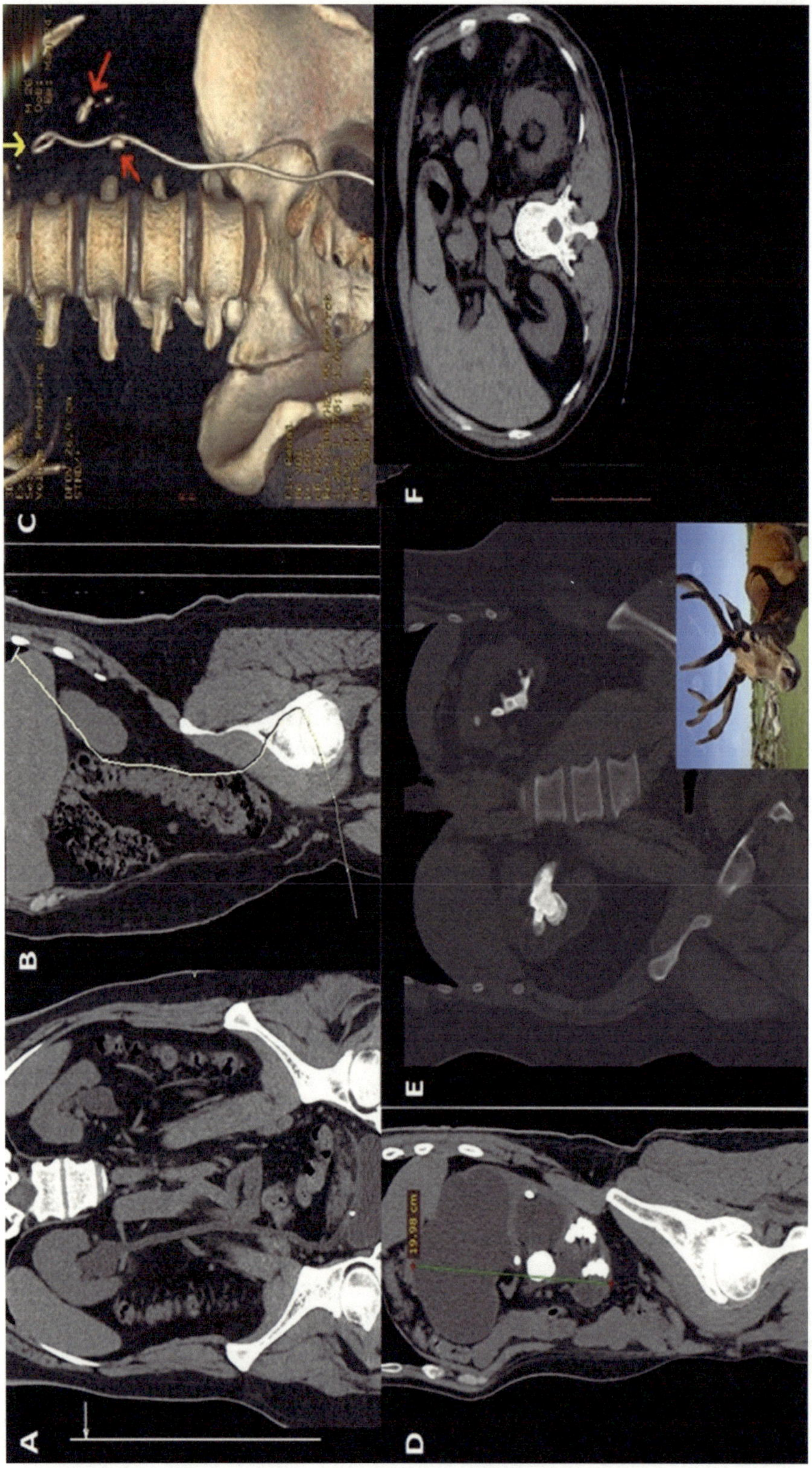

Figure 14.
CT photomontage. A and B: curved planar reformat to delineate the anatomy of the ureter with hyper dense calculus seen in the right distal ureter. C: volume-rendered CT shows the DJ stent. D: sagittal CT scan for assessing the length of kidney. E: bilateral staghorn calculi with inset displaying name origin. F: axial CT shows left hydronephrosis and peri – nephric fat stranding.

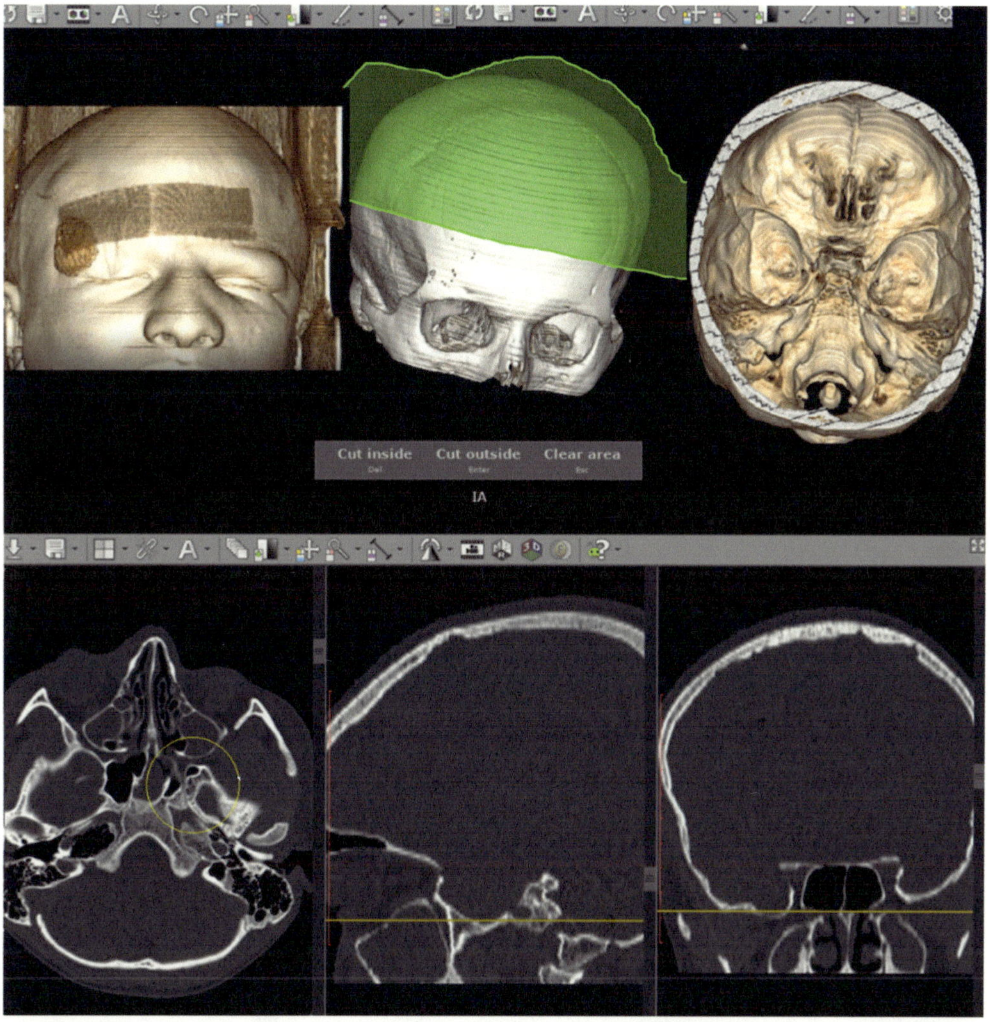

Figure 15.
Skull base cross sectional and surface anatomy on 2D and 3D CT; 3D manipulation tools (virtual scalpel, rotator) allow the operator to pan, rotate, zoom, and images.

Advanced MDCT 64 and 128-slice scanners help in hollow tube examination via shaded surface display. Virtual colonoscopy, also known as computed tomographic colonoscopy (CTC), is now being used in screening colorectal malignancies. It has sensitivity nearly equal to optical colonoscopy. Virtual bronchoscopy is a diagnostic technique that produces high-resolution images of the tracheobronchial tree via minimum intensity projection (MinP) (**Figure 16**). [87–89]

Dual-energy CT is a new technology that utilizes two X-ray tubes in the gantry instead of one and has vast advantages over MDCT, for example, characterization of renal calculi, cysts, masses, differentiation of iodine extravasation from hemorrhage, etc. [90]

Tomotherapy is an advanced form of therapy that combines intensity-modulated therapy with CT scan precision in radiation oncology. CT is used for contouring in stereotactic radiosurgery for precise localization of tumors (**Figure 17**). [91]

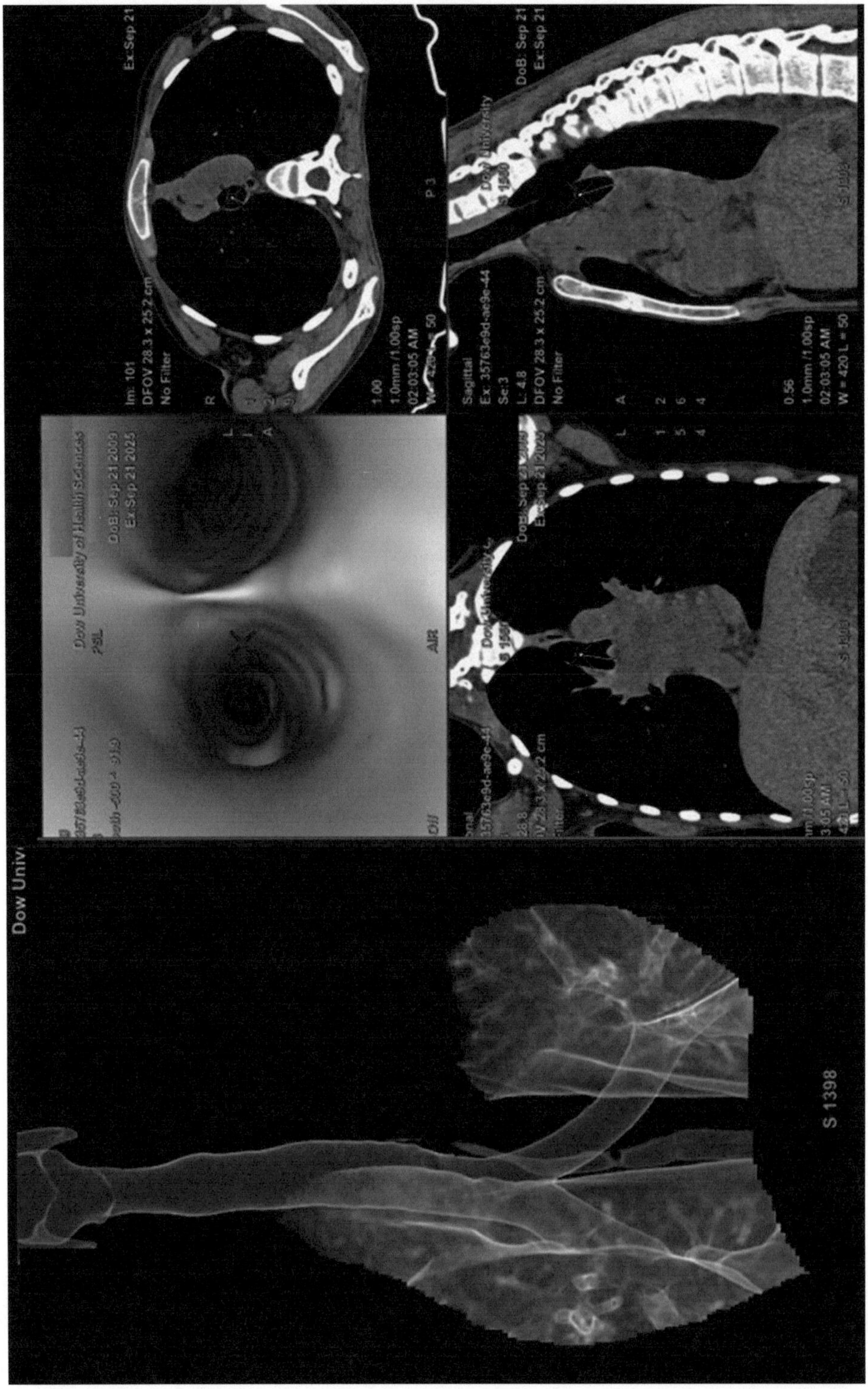

Figure 16.
CT virtual bronchoscopy (projection and source images) of a adult.

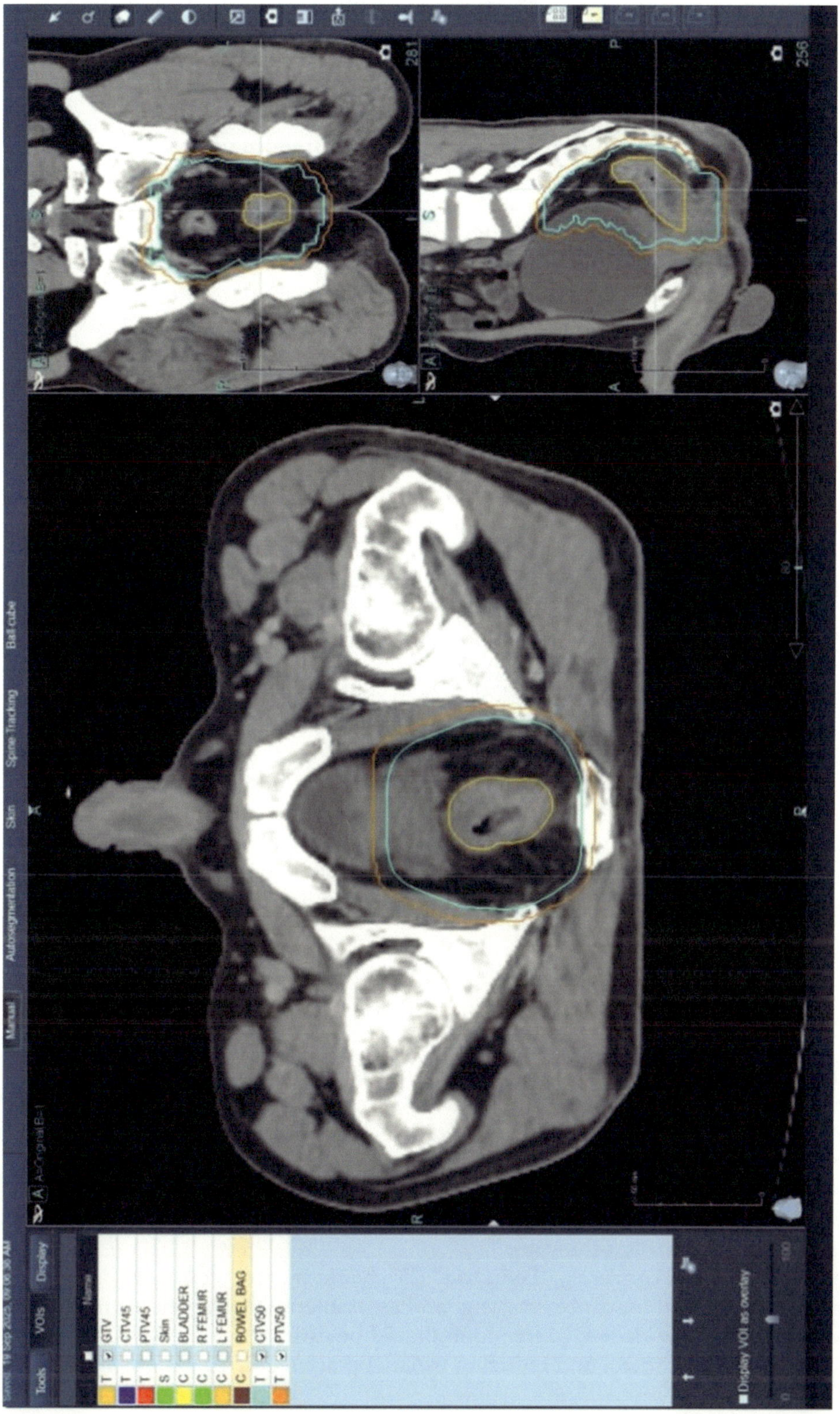

Figure 17.
Tomotherapy contouring in a case of rectal carcinoma. multi planar CT images showing the of colored lines representing gross tumor volume (GTV), clinical target volume (CTV), and planning target volume (PTV). Image courtesy: Dr. Aneeta Ghulam Ali, Department of CyberKnife and Tomotherapy, JPMC, Pakistan.

CT fluoroscopy combines cross-sectional imaging with the movement and tracking perception of fluoroscopy. It is essential for image-guided biopsies and interventions, including trans-arterial chemo embolization and radio frequency ablation [90]. While bone mineral density is routinely assessed via DEXA scan, a CT scan can assess bone density subjectively but also quantitatively – a novel concept for opportunistic screening of osteoporosis (**Figure 18**) [92].

Tumor heterogeneity can be quantified into mineable data via radiomics – a new advancement in radiology. In one study, computed tomography texture analysis (CTTA) was used to predict the breast cancer histo-pathological features and found no statistically significant differences (**Figure 19**) [93].

CT lung cancer screening is recommended for adults who are at high risk of developing the disease due to their smoking history and age [94].

Dental Cone Beam CT is a special type of 3D X-ray equipment used when plain facial or dental X-rays are not sufficient. It is utilized in orthodontics, ENT, dental implantology, and oral and maxillofacial radiology [95].

Photon counting CT is a new CT technology recently approved by the FDA. It uses a semiconductor rather than a scintillator to generate electronic signals in the detector. It has a few advantages over conventional CT, for example, improved spatial resolution, reduced dose, and fewer artifacts [96].

Artificial intelligence (AI), including deep learning (DL) and machine learning (ML), is revolutionizing modern healthcare by enhancing diagnostic capabilities in both trauma care and precision oncology. In the emergency department, AI-powered systems analyze radiological images like CT scans to rapidly and accurately detect subtle and often life-threatening pathologies in traumatic brain and abdominal injuries, significantly improving the speed and precision of diagnostic interpretation [97, 98]. Furthermore, AI and ML facilitate advanced data analysis in cancer care, extracting rich quantitative data from medical images to enable detailed tumor pheno-typing and support the development of highly personalized precision care strategies.

From an economic perspective, CT has opened new doors for radiologists' employment, including Tele-radiology and the worldwide trading of machine components.

14. Imaging appropriateness and low dose CT techniques

CT has been the major source of ionizing radiation, which has the potential to induce carcinogenesis. ACR Appropriateness Criteria help referring doctors recommend appropriate imaging for a specific clinical condition. There have been rising concerns regarding the inappropriate use of CT. In one study conducted in Pakistan on 1,206 HRCT chest scans, 44.6% of scans were found to be inappropriate! Each and every imaging study must be justified, considering the ALARA principle, i.e., "as low as reasonably achievable".

Because of similar concerns, "Pediatric" CT should be reserved only for cardiovascular anomalies, cancer staging, and assessment of complex trauma/non-accidental injury. Low-dose CT technique should be utilized for CT KUB, including automatic exposure control and reducing mAs/kVp according to patient size [99–103].

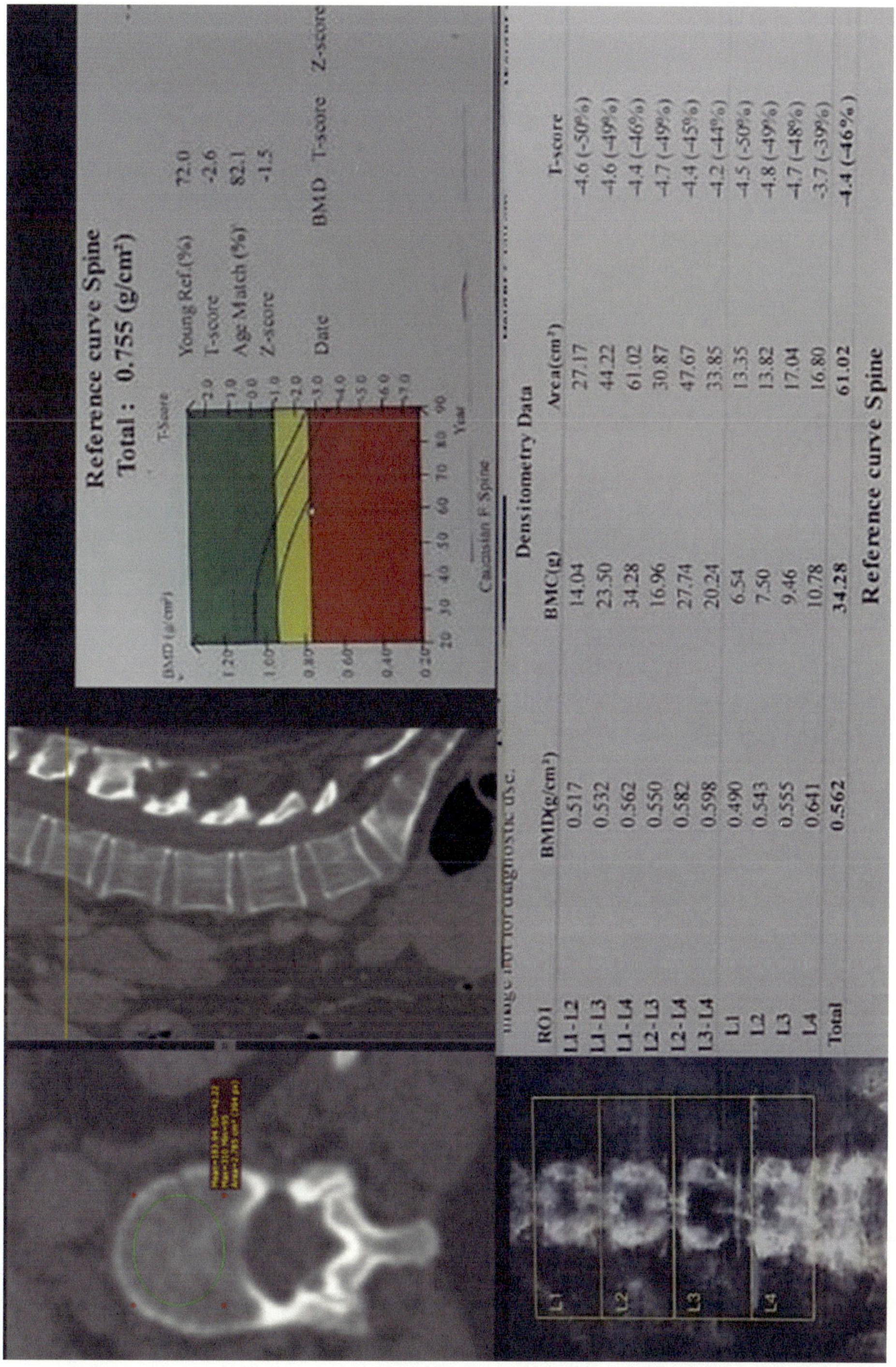

Figure 18.
Utility of CT scan via HU measurements for assessing bone density.

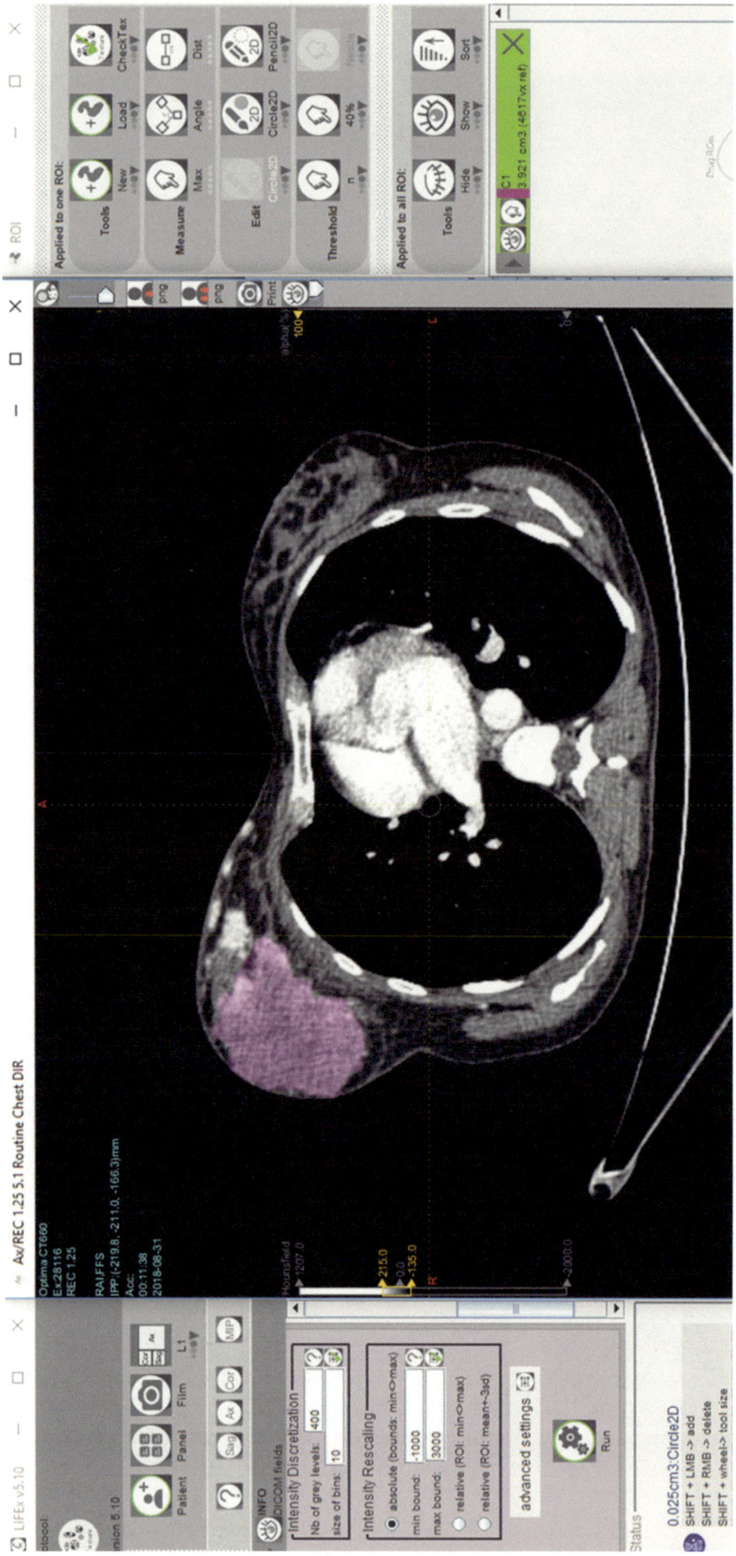

Figure 19.
Display of CTTA processing in radiomics software. Region of interest drawn over the lesion.

To avoid unnecessary radiation exposure due to a CT scan, in trauma patients, the Canadian CT Head Rule in an emergency department provides an approach for physicians to evaluate the appropriate use of CT scans in patients with minor head injuries and those over 16 years old with blunt head trauma [104].

Although radiation is a concern in the pediatric population, the risk of missed injury often outweighs the potential radiation harm. Using a multidisciplinary approach, specialist interpretation, and structured imaging protocols, including the use of low-dose CT scans, helps reduce the radiation dose.

Acknowledgement

Authors are grateful to Dr. Sami Khan, Basildon University Hospital, UK, and Dr. Aneeta Ghulam Ali, Diagnostic Radiologist, JPMC, Pakistan, for sharing Virtual Dissection and cyber knife experience, respectively, and Dr. Nida Ihsan, PET CT Diagnostic Radiologist, JPMC, Pakistan, for providing patient data in **Figure 12**.

The author acknowledges the use of Trinka AI grammar checker for language polishing of the manuscript.

Conflict of interest

Author declares no conflict of interest.

Authors' contribution

MH and JV were involved in the designing, preparation, and editing of the manuscript, as well as the literature search.

Abbreviation

AI	Artificial Intelligence
ABPA	Allergic Bronchopulmonary Aspergillosis
ACR	American College of Radiology
CXR	Chest X-ray
DJ	Double J stent
FDA	Food and Drug Administration
FESS	Functional Endoscopic Sinus Surgery
IT	Information Technology
KUB	Kidneys, Ureters, and Bladder
kVp	Kilo volt peak
mAs	milliampere second
MDCT	Multi detector CT
MPR	Multi planar reformat
NICE	National Institute for Health and Care Excellence
TNM	Tumor, Node, and Metastasis
VD	Virtual Dissection

Author details

Mahnoor Hafeez[1*] and Javerya Sattar[2]

1 Senior Instructor & Consultant Radiologist, Dow Institute of Radiology, Dow University of Health Sciences, Karachi, Pakistan

2 Senior Registrar & Consultant Radiologist, Dow Institute of Radiology, Dow University of Health Sciences, Karachi, Pakistan

*Address all correspondence to: mahnoor.hafeez@yahoo.com

References

[1] Nadgir R, Yousem DM. Neuroradiology: The Requisites E-book. Elsevier Health Sciences; 2016

[2] Bushong SC. Radiologic science for technologists. Physics, Biology, and Protection. 1984;**9**

[3] Hammer M. XRay Physics. Interactive Radiology Physics. 2013. Available from: http://xrayphysics.com/ctsim.html

[4] Penelope J, Allisy-roberts W. Farr's Physics for Medical Imaging. INDIA: ELSEVIER; 2008

[5] Hafeez M, Comparing effective doses in plain abdominal CT scans between two scanners of the institute. 2022

[6] Wintermark M, et al. Imaging recommendations for acute stroke and transient ischemic attack patients: A joint statement by the American Society of Neuroradiology, the American College of Radiology, and the Society of NeuroInterventional Surgery. American Journal of Neuroradiology. 2013;**34**:E117–E127

[7] Zhang X, et al. Global, regional, and national burden of stroke attributable to diet high in sodium from 1990 to 2019: A systematic analysis from the global burden of disease study 2019. Frontiers in Neurology. 2024;**15**:1437633

[8] Akbarzadeh MA, et al. Role of imaging in early diagnosis of acute ischemic stroke: A literature review. The Egyptian Journal of Neurology, Psychiatry and Neurosurgery 2021;**57**:175

[9] Goyal M, Ospel J. Challenges to stroke care 5 years after endovascular therapy became the standard. The Lancet Neurology. 2020;**19**(3):210–211

[10] Hacke W. Thrombolysis with alteplase 3 to 4.5 hours after acute ischemic stroke. New England Journal of Medicine. 2007;**358**:1327

[11] Korb PJ, Jones W. Coding in stroke and other cerebrovascular diseases. Continuum. 2017;**23**(1):e1–e11

[12] Hoang JK, et al. Imaging thyroid disease: Updates, imaging approach, and management pearls. Radiologic Clinics of North America. 2015;**53**:145–161

[13] Kanematsu M, et al. Hepatocellular carcinoma: The role of helical biphasic contrast-enhanced CT versus CT during arterial portography. Radiology. 1997;**205**:75–80

[14] Wang X, et al. Impact of the Alberta Stroke Program CT Score subregions on long-term functional outcomes in acute ischemic stroke: Results from two multicenter studies in China. Journal of Translational Internal Medicine. 2024;**12**:197–208

[15] Sutton D, A textbook of radiology and imaging. 1987

[16] Chin R, Nguyen T. Synchronous malignant otitis externa and squamous cell carcinoma of the external auditory canal. Case Reports in Otolaryngology. 2013;**2013**(1)

[17] Farhan N, et al. Identification of significant anatomical variations in the nose and anterior skull base using computed tomography: A cross-sectional study. Cureus. 2020;12(6)

[18] Abbasi H, et al. Diagnostic accuracy of CT PNS in diagnosing fungal sinusitis and its relation with endoscopy and histopathological findings. Age (Mean & SD). 2023;**39**:705

[19] Weerakkody Y, Knipe H, Walizai T. Radiopaedia.org. Chronic sinusitis. 2014

[20] Nazir R, et al. Understanding Hemifacial Microsomia: Correlation of CT and clinical findings. Pakistan Journal of Radiology. 2016;**26**(3)

[21] Hafeez M. The constellation of centronuclear myopathy and craniofacial dysmorphism. Pakistan Journal of Neurological Sciences (PJNS). 2021;**16**(4):25–27

[22] Khan AA, Hafeez M. The Constellation Of Craniofacial And Cns Anomalies In A Single Patient. Pakistan Journal of Radiology. 2017;**27**(3)

[23] Melikian N, et al. Fractional flow reserve and myocardial perfusion imaging in patients with angiographic multivessel coronary artery disease. JACC: Cardiovascular Interventions. 2010;**3**:307–314

[24] Bilchick KC, et al. Effectiveness of integrating delayed computed tomography angiography imaging for left atrial appendage thrombus exclusion into the care of patients undergoing ablation of atrial fibrillation. Heart Rhythm. 2016;**13**:12–19

[25] Mahabbah MN, Rafsanjani R, Putri BA. The analysis study of diagnostic imaging performance and accuracy of congestive heart failure: A comprehensive systematic review. The Indonesian Journal of General Medicine. 2025;**9**(2):1–19

[26] Siddique U, et al. Imaging road-map for CTA coronary reporting: Post processing mdct techniques in diagnosing severity of coronary artery disease. Pakistan Journal of Radiology. 2024;**34**(4)

[27] Alam S, et al. CT radiation dose reduction in pediatric cardiovascular anomalies–clinical audit in a single centre. Pakistan Journal of Radiology. 2017;**27**(3)

[28] Khan AA, Hafeez M. The asymptomatic dissecting aortic aneurysm: An incidental finding on CT. Journal of the College of Physicians and Surgeons Pakistan. 2018;**28**(6):482–485

[29] Hafeez M, Sattar A. Diagnostic accuracy of Non-ECG gated chest CT (NEGCT) for cardiac chambers' dimensions in comparison with echocardiography: Non-ECG gated chest CT (NEGCT) for cardiac chambers' dimensions. Journal of Fatima Jinnah Medical University. 2022;**16**(2):53–57

[30] Hafeez M, Sattar A, Naz N. The accuracy and precision of plain CT chest for diagnosis of anaemia. JPMA: The Journal of the Pakistan Medical Association. 2024;**74**(9):1593–1597

[31] Saade C, et al. Impact of various iodine concentrations of iohexol and iodixanol contrast media on image reconstruction techniques in a vascular-specific contrast media phantom: Quantitative and qualitative image quality assessment. La Radiologia Medica. 2021;**126**:221–230

[32] Bhatla N, et al. Revised FIGO staging for carcinoma of the cervix uteri. International Journal of Gynecology & Obstetrics. 2019;**145**:129–135

[33] on Thoracic EP, et al. ACR appropriateness criteria® staging and follow-up of esophageal cancer. Journal of the American College of Radiology. 2022;**19**:S462–S472

[34] Sumi M, Ohki M, Nakamura T. Comparison of sonography and CT for differentiating benign from malignant cervical lymph nodes in patients with squamous cell carcinoma of the head and neck. American Journal of Roentgenology. 2001;**176**(4): 1019–1024

[35] Rasheed W, et al. Diagnostic accuracy of high-resolution computed tomography of chest in diagnosing sputum smear positive and sputum smear negative pulmonary tuberculosis. Cureus 2020. 12(6)

[36] Aramini B, et al. Giant bulla or pneumothorax: How to distinguish. International Journal of Surgery Case Reports. 2019;**62**:21–23

[37] Block J, Jordanov MI, Stack LB, Thurman RJ. Atlas of Emergency Radiology. McGraw Hill Professional; 2013

[38] Ajlan AM, et al. Detectability of choledocholithiasis on CT: The effect of positive intraduodenal enteric contrast on portovenous contrast-enhanced studies. Saudi Journal of Gastroenterology. 2015;**21**:306–312

[39] Rodgers SK, et al. Imaging after cesarean delivery: Acute and chronic complications. Radiographics. 2012;**32**:1693–1712

[40] Tan CH, et al. Pathways of extrapelvic spread of pelvic disease: Imaging findings. Radiographics. 2011;**31**:117–133

[41] Pescatori LC, et al. Clinical impact of computed tomography in the emergency department in nontraumatic chest and abdominal conditions. Emergency Radiology. 2018;**25**:393–398

[42] Iacobellis F, et al. Current standards for and clinical impact of emergency radiology in major trauma. International Journal of Environmental Research and Public Health. 2022;**19**:539

[43] Wirth S, et al. European society of emergency radiology: Guideline on radiological polytrauma imaging and service (short version). Insights Into Imaging. 2020;**11**:135

[44] Cimbanassi S, Chiara O. Diagnostic protocols in trauma care, in trauma centers and acute care surgery: A novel organizational and cultural model. Springer; 2021. p. 45–57

[45] Hakim W, et al. Trauma whole-body MDCT: An assessment of image quality in conventional dual-phase and modified biphasic injection. The British Journal of Radiology. 2016;**89**(1063):20160160

[46] Leung V, et al. Implementation of a split-bolus single-pass CT protocol at a UK major trauma centre to reduce excess radiation dose in trauma pan-CT. Clinical Radiology. 2015;**70**:1110–1115

[47] Maheshwari E, et al. Split-bolus MDCT urography: Upper tract opacification and performance for

upper tract tumors in patients with hematuria. American Journal of Roentgenology. 2010;**194**:453–458

[48] Iacobellis F, et al. Dual-phase CT for the assessment of acute vascular injuries in high-energy blunt trauma: The imaging findings and management implications. The British Journal of Radiology. 2016;**89**(1061)

[49] Murao S, et al. Effect of earlier door-to-CT and door-to-bleeding control in severe blunt trauma: A retrospective cohort study. Journal of Clinical Medicine. 2021;**10**:1522

[50] Mirvis SE, Shanmuganathan K. Trauma radiology: Part IV. Imaging of acute craniocerebral trauma. Journal of Intensive Care Medicine. 1994;**9** (6):305–315

[51] Poletti P-A, et al. Traumatic injuries: Role of imaging in the management of the polytrauma victim (conservative expectation). European Radiology. 2002;**12**:969–978

[52] Heiken JP, Katz DS, Menu Y. Emergency radiology of the abdomen and pelvis: Imaging of the non-traumatic and traumatic acute abdomen. Diseases of the Abdomen and Pelvis 2018-2021: Diagnostic Imaging-IDKD Book. 2018;123–143

[53] Colleran GC, et al. ESR Essentials: Imaging of suspected child abuse—practice recommendations by the European Society of Paediatric Radiology. European Radiology. 2025;**35**:1868–1880

[54] Schermerhorn SM, Muensterer OJ, Ignacio Jr RC. Identification and evaluation of non-accidental trauma in the pediatric population: A clinical review. Children. 2024;**11**(4):413

[55] Patel H, et al. Fat stranding associated with high-grade colon adenocarcinoma: A case report. Cureus. 2024;**16**(4)

[56] Hafeez M, Sattar A. Contributions and challenges of radiology in the era of COVID-19 pandemic. Journal of the College of Physicians and Surgeons Pakistan. 2020;**30**:84

[57] Thornton E, et al. Patterns of fat stranding. American Journal of Roentgenology. 2011;**197**:W1–W14

[58] Raman SP, Fishman EK. Advances in CT imaging of GI malignancies. Gastrointestinal Cancer Research: GCR. 2012;**5**(3 Suppl 1):S4

[59] Rice TW, Patil DT, Blackstone EH. AJCC/UICC staging of cancers of the esophagus and esophagogastric junction: Application to clinical practice. Annals of Cardiothoracic Surgery. 2017;**6**(2):119

[60] Becker M, Zaidi H. Imaging in head and neck squamous cell carcinoma: The potential role of PET/MRI. The British Journal of Radiology. 2014;**87**(1036)

[61] Naz N, Sattar J, Ashrafi SK. Diagnostic accuracy of computed tomography in detecting bone invasion due to squamous cell carcinoma of buccal mucosa. Journal of the College of Physicians and Surgeons Pakistan. 2018;**28**(11):829–833

[62] Detterbeck FC, et al. The eighth edition lung cancer stage classification. Chest. 2017;**151**:193–203

[63] Shetty A, Hacking C, Sharma R. et al. Positron emission tomography. Reference article, Radiopaedia.org.

DOI: 10.53347/rID-29716 [Accessed: 2026-January-20]

[64] Wang X. PET/CT: Appropriate application in lymphoma. Chinese Clinical Oncology. 2015;**4**(1):4–4

[65] Ur Rehman MH & Khan AA. The ct criteria of unresectability for pancreatic carcinoma. Pakistan Journal of Radiology. 2017;**27**(2): Available from: https://www.pakjr.com/index.php/PJR/article/view/588

[66] Tamm EP, et al. State-of-the-art imaging of pancreatic neuroendocrine tumors. Surgical Oncology Clinics of North America. 2016;**25**:375–400

[67] Martin J, et al. Colorectal liver metastases: Current management and future perspectives. World Journal of Clinical Oncology. 2020;**11**:761

[68] Hazhirkarzar B, et al. Current state of the art imaging approaches for colorectal liver metastasis. Hepatobiliary Surgery and Nutrition. 2020;**9**:35

[69] Tsili AC, Argyropoulou MI. Advances of multidetector computed tomography in the characterization and staging of renal cell carcinoma. World Journal of Radiology. 2015; 7(6):110

[70] Sehnal B, et al. New FIGO 2023 staging system of endometrial cancer: An updated review on a current hot topic. Geburtshilfe Und Frauenheilkunde. 2025

[71] Witjes JA, et al. EAU guidelines on muscle-invasive and metastatic bladder cancer: Summary of the 2013 guidelines. European Urology. 2014;**65**:778–792

[72] Flicek K, et al. Correlation of radiologic with surgical peritoneal cancer index scores in patients with pseudomyxoma peritonei and peritoneal carcinomatosis: How well can we predict resectability? Journal of Gastrointestinal Surgery. 2016;**20**:307–312

[73] Fallon EA, et al. Peritoneal cancer index correlates with radiographic assessment of colorectal carcinomatosis. Annals of Surgical Oncology. 2024;1–9

[74] Rafiq N, et al. Utility of unenhanced CT KUB: Beyond urolithiasis. Annals Of Abbasi Shaheed Hospital And Karachi Medical & Dental College. 2023;**28**:45–52

[75] Farooq Z, et al. An audit of radiological investigation in acute renal colic as well as diagnostic yield of CT KUB in terms of renal calculi and alternative diagnosis. Pakistan Journal of Radiology. 2024;**34**(4)

[76] Sattar A, Hafeez M. Efficacy of plain computed tomography (CT) abdomen for urinary stone disease in symptomatic patients. Methodology. 2020

[77] Reimer RP, et al. Manual kidney stone size measurements in computed tomography are most accurate using multiplanar image reformatations and bone window settings. Scientific Reports. 2021;**11**(1)

[78] Rasheed Y, et al. Extracorporeal Shock Wave Lithotripsy (ESWL) outcome based on CT scan and patient parameters using ESWL score. Journal of the College of Physicians and Surgeons–Pakistan: JCPSP. 2023;**33**: 199–204

[79] Khaliq DM, Faiq SM, Jesrani AK. Effect of CT scan hounsfield units (attenuation value of stones) in predicting outcomes of ESWL in renal calculi, experience at SIUT. Pakistan Journal of Radiology. 2021;**31**(3)

[80] Sindhi Y, et al. Extracorporeal shockwave lithotripsy versus ureteroscopy: A first line distal ureteric stone treatment. Pakistan Journal of Medicine and Dentistry. 2021;**10**:49–54

[81] Arshad S, et al. Significance of hounsfield units on non-contrast computed tomography in determining stone free rate after ESWL. Pakistan Journal of Radiology. 2018;**28**(2)

[82] O'Donnell C, Woodford N. Post-mortem radiology—a new sub-speciality? Clinical Radiology. 2008;**63**(11):1189–1194

[83] Sohail S, Mirza FH, Khan QS. Postmortem computed tomography for diagnosis of cause of death in male prisoners. JPMA: The Journal of the Pakistan Medical Association. 2010;**60**(1):4

[84] Furlow B. CT-Guided interventional radiology. Radiologic Technology. 2019;**90**(6)

[85] Hafeez M, et al., the innovation of skull base virtual dissection in Medical College. Available at SSRN 5165020

[86] Sami K. 'Virtual Dissection'. Scientific Session, 54th Annual Medical Symposium. Najamuddin Auditorium. Jinnah Postgraduate Medical Centre (JPMC), Pakistan; 2019

[87] Saglam M, Ors F. Virtual colonoscopy: Indications, techniques, findings. In: Endoscopic Procedures in Colon and Rectum. IntechOpen; 2011

[88] Ganeshan D, Elsayes KM, Vining D. Virtual colonoscopy: Utility, impact and overview. World Journal of Radiology. 2013;**5**(3):61

[89] Horton KM, Horton MR, Fishman EK. Advanced visualization of airways with 64-MDCT: 3D mapping and virtual bronchoscopy. American Journal of Roentgenology. 2007;**189**(6):1387–1396

[90] Drew Z, Walizai T, Campos A et al. CT fluoroscopy. Reference article. Radiopaedia.org. DOI: 10.53347/rID-62860 [Accessed: 2026-January-20]

[91] Welsh JS, et al. Helical tomotherapy: An innovative technology and approach to radiation therapy. Technology in Cancer Research & Treatment. 2002;**1**:311–316

[92] Elarjani T, et al. Quantifying bone quality using computed tomography Hounsfield units in the mid-sagittal view of the lumbar spine. World Neurosurgery. 2021;**151**:e418–e425

[93] Hafeez M, Rahim A, Awais M, Sattar A. CT texture analysis (CTTA) parameters as imaging biomarkers for predicting histopathological and molecular features of carcinoma. Clinical Radiology. 2020;**75**:e2 DOI: 10.1016/j.crad.2020.11.011

[94] Screening for lung cancer. Lung Cancer, [Accessed: 2024-October-15] Available from: https://www.cdc.gov/lung- cancer/screening/index.html

[95] Knipe H, Raymond Chieng S, Bell D, et al Cone-beam CT. Reference article, Radiopaedia.org. [Accessed: 2026-January-16] DOI: 10.53347/rID-46277

[96] Esquivel A, et al. Photon-counting detector CT: Key points radiologists should know. Korean Journal of Radiology. 2022;**23**:854

[97] Bellal M, et al. A Comprehensive Survey on Deep Learning in Abdominal Imaging: Datasets, Techniques, and Performance Metrics. IEEE Access; 2025

[98] de la Rosa E, et al. A radiomics approach to traumatic brain injury prediction in CT scans. 2019 IEEE 16th International Symposium on Biomedical Imaging (ISBI 2019). 2019. IEEE

[99] Forman HP, et al. Masters of radiology panel discussion: Who is accountable for the appropriateness of studies—the radiologist, the referring physician, or both? American Journal of Roentgenology. 2010;**195**:968–973

[100] Ebdon-Jackson S, Frija G, Radiology ESO. Improving justification of medical exposures using ionising radiation: Considerations and approaches from the European Society of Radiology. Insights into Imaging. 2021;**12**(1):2

[101] Sattar A, et al. Appropriateness and clinical outcome of chest computed tomography without intravenous contrast: A study conducted in Pakistan. Respiratory Investigation. 2018;**56**: 342–348

[102] McCollough CH, et al. Strategies for reducing radiation dose in CT. Radiologic Clinics of North America. 2009;**47**:27

[103] Anwar M, et al. Comparative diagnostic accuracy of low-dose CT Kub and conventional CT in detecting renal and ureteric Calculi. Pakistan Journal of Medical & Health Sciences. 2023;**17**:283–283

[104] Reddy A, et al. Efficacy of the Canadian CT head rule in patients presenting to the emergency department with minor head injury. Indian Journal of Critical Care Medicine: Peer-reviewed, Official Publication of Indian Society of Critical Care Medicine. 2024;**28**:148

Chapter 4

Venous Invasion in Hepatocellular Carcinoma - CT

Youstina Elamir and Mai Ashraf Saad Zaghloul

Abstract

Hepatocellular carcinoma is characterized by its strong propensity for invasion of vascular structures, mainly the portal vein and, uncommonly, the hepatic veins and inferior vena cava (IVC). Differentiating malignant from bland thrombus is crucial in determining the therapeutic approach, as the presence of malignant venous invasion is considered an advanced stage with limited therapeutic options and poorer prognosis. Adequate triphasic computed tomography (CT) is important in the detection of macrovascular venous invasion and in assessing the extent of malignant thrombus. Features of malignant thrombus include expansion of the vein, enhancement, internal neovascularity, direct continuity with the HCC mass, and showing a similar pattern to that of HCC. The presence of large malignant thrombus can cause significant hemodynamic changes in the liver; also, large malignant portal venous thrombus (PVTT) can cause portal hypertension, gastrointestinal bleeding, and might lead to multiple intrahepatic tumor seeding and recurrence. Involvement of the inferior vena cava by tumor thrombus and the right atrium can lead to secondary Budd–Chiari syndrome, pulmonary embolism, pulmonary metastases, and immediate death if the malignant thrombus infiltrates the heart. Determining the extent of malignant thrombus is important in choosing the appropriate management, whether hepatic resection if the thrombus is limited or systemic therapy in advanced cases. Missing venous invasion has a great negative impact on patient management; causes of missing it include inadequate imaging, similar patterns of malignant thrombus to the primary tumor, forgetting to revise hepatic veins and IVC (which is not usually written in templates), and doctor exhaustion.

Keywords: hepatocellular carcinoma, computed tomography (CT), malignant venous thrombosis, portal vein, inferior vena cava

1. Introduction

Hepatocellular carcinoma (HCC) is the most common primary malignant tumor affecting the liver, usually seen in a cirrhotic liver.

It is considered the fifth most common cancer and also the second most common cause of cancer death [1]. HCC has a great tendency to invade major vascular structures, such as the portal vein (PV), less commonly the hepatic vein (HV), and the inferior vena cava (IVC) [2].

Tumor thrombus invading the hepatic vein (HV) to extend to the inferior vena cava (IVC) and right atrium (RA) has also been reported [3, 4].

Neoplastic and bland thrombi are formed through different pathophysiological mechanisms with different prognoses. Bland thrombus, which results from the slow flow of portal blood, consists of clotted blood or fibrin with no viable cells [5]. The bland thrombus might be resolved following thrombolytic and anticoagulant treatment, unlike malignant invasion, which is typically induced by the direct invasion of hepatocellular carcinoma (HCC) into the vein, usually the portal vein (PV) [6]. It is most often associated with earlier recurrence and metastasis in the liver, even following surgical resection [7, 8] Detection of malignant thrombosis is challenging, as it is asymptomatic in many patients. It might be detected during either routine staging or follow-up imaging [9].

Vascular invasion in HCC can be macrovascular invasion, typically visualized as invasion of the portal or hepatic venous system, or microvascular invasion, defined as microscopic infiltration of small vascular channels; both are key determinants of prognosis [10, 11].

Macrovascular invasion can be readily identified on cross-sectional imaging and usually precludes curative therapeutic options like partial hepatectomy or liver transplantation. In contrast, microvascular invasion is detectable only on histopathological examination, making it difficult to predict preoperatively despite advances in imaging biomarkers [10, 11].

2. Differentiating malignant from bland thrombus

The presence of malignant thrombus is considered a high stage with limited therapeutic chances (**Table 1**). Therefore, differentiating bland from malignant thrombus is very significant in assessing therapeutic options and predicting survival [12].

Adequate imaging is crucial for diagnosing or excluding the presence of venous thrombosis. Owing to the higher risk of venous thrombosis in cancer patients, the limited reliability of clinical signs, along with other clinical indicators such as D-dimer, cannot be interpreted in patients diagnosed with cancer [13].

Differentiating malignant from bland thrombus is important for the management of the patient. CT and MRI are very useful in detecting malignant thrombus and characterizing its extent [14].

Imaging Features	Malignant thrombus	Bland thrombus
Expansion of the vein	Present	Not present
Similar features to HCC	Present	Not present
Enhancement	Present	Not present
Direct continuity with the primary	Present	Not present
Internal neovascularity	Present	Not present

Table 1.
Differentiation between malignant and bland thrombus.

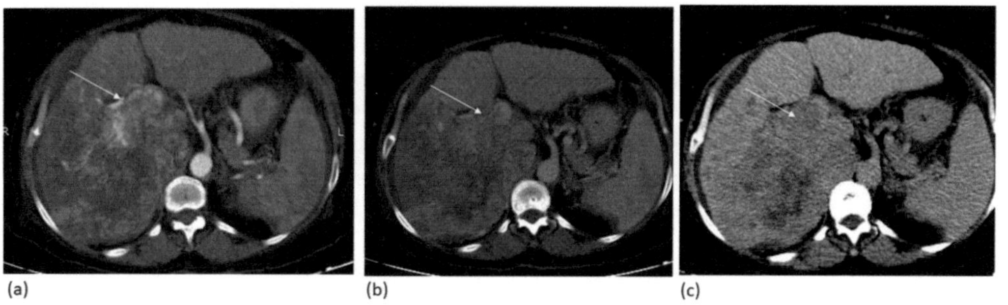

(a) (b) (c)

Figure 1.
Axial triphasic study for an HCC case showing expansion of the portal vein, demonstrating similar features to the primary tumor in the form of arterial hyperenhancement (a) and wash out in the later phases (b, c), with internal neovascularity (a).

It is important for the detection of either tumoral or benign thrombus on CT to consider an adequate bolus of contrast to ensure optimal opacification of the vessels [15].

Malignant thrombus shows expansion of the vein, while bland thrombus. Malignant thrombus shows enhancement, but bland thrombus often appears as a filling defect and doesn't enhance. Malignant thrombus shows direct continuity from the primary tumor, while bland thrombus does not. Malignant thrombus shows similar features to the primary tumor, while bland thrombus does not [16]. The pattern of enhancement in malignant thrombus may resemble that of the primary malignancy, including hyperenhancement in the arterial phase and washout in the delayed phase in HCC cases [9].

The detection of neovascularity within a portal vein thrombus on CT scans has been documented to exhibit 100% specificity for malignancy (**Figure 1**) [17].

Shunts can be associated with tumor thrombus and may result in transient hepatic attenuation differences (THAD) [18].

Differentiating malignant and benign thrombi can also be done by 18 F-fluorodeoxyglucose (FDG) positron emission tomography/CT, as malignant thrombi show higher FDG uptake than bland thrombi [19, 20].

In MRI, malignant thrombi typically demonstrate restricted diffusion, whereas bland thrombi show no or minimal restriction. Additionally, T2-weighted imaging demonstrates intermediate signal intensity of the malignant thrombus, while bland thrombus shows low signal intensity [16].

3. CT imaging

The most important requirement for proper visualization of venous thrombosis at CT is an adequate bolus of contrast for sufficient vessel opacification. In routine staging or restaging CT, 100 mL of IV contrast doses are usually used [21].

Triphasic CT is required to image the entire liver in the arterial, portal, and delayed phases.

Non-enhanced CT (NECT) is usually performed before contrast injection to differentiate actual enhancement from hyperdense lesions, especially post-transarterial chemoembolization in HCC cases, and can detect calcification that might be observed in chronic bland thrombus.

Late arterial phase, usually acquired 30–35 seconds post-injection, is useful for the detection of neovascularity and enhancement of the malignant venous thrombus.

Portal phase is usually acquired 60–70 seconds post-injection, which is the best phase for assessment of opacification of the venous structures, but sometimes a flow artifact may cause misinterpretation, mistaking it for actual thrombosis.

Delayed phase is usually acquired 3–5 minutes post-injection and is useful for differentiating flow artifacts from actual thrombosis. It also shows the washout of malignant venous invasion as the primary in cases of HCC.

In some studies, dual-energy spectral computed tomography (DESCT) demonstrated greater precision in distinguishing between bland and tumor thrombus compared to a conventional CT scan with contrast [12, 22–24].

The latest DESCT imaging technology enables the spectral differentiation and quantification of materials within the object. In cases with contrast images, material decomposition effectively separates the signal from iodinated contrast from that of the soft tissue, resulting in a series of iodine-based images that offer insights into the distribution of the contrast material within the organ [25, 26].

The phase of the portal vein is usually selected for examining portal vein thrombosis, not only because thrombi are more readily detected during this phase, but also because their connections with primary hepatic lesions (if present) are more evident compared to other phases [12].

But DESCT is usually not done in routine staging or follow-up imaging; triphasic CT imaging remains the primary method of investigation.

4. Venous invasion

4.1 Portal vein invasion

Hepatocellular carcinoma (HCC) is considered the most common cause of bland or malignant portal vein thrombosis (PVTT) [27].

PVTT is the most common type of macrovascular invasion in HCC, with its diagnostic occurrence ranging from 10% to over 40% [28, 29–30].

The presence of malignant thrombus is an important determinant of tumor staging and prognosis and affects treatment selection. Portal vein invasion in HCC renders the patient unsuitable for surgical resection, orthotopic liver transplantation, and chemoembolization, owing to the high incidence of tumor recurrence and lower survival associated with these patients [31].

It can be identified by a triphasic contrast CT study, where it appears as solid lesions within the portal vein throughout all phases. The PVTT shows arterial phase enhancement and washout in the delayed phase [32].

In contrast, bland thrombus of the portal vein (PVT) frequently occurs due to complications associated with cirrhosis or splenectomy. There is no enhancement in the arterial phase and it can be treated with anticoagulant therapy. Precisely distinguishing malignant portal vein thrombosis from bland thrombus is crucial [33].

HCC can show either a massive, nodular, or infiltrative pattern. The presence of tumor thrombus in both massive and nodular patterns of HCC can be detected through imaging by its continuity with the tumor and the pattern of enhancement, like that of HCC, in the form of arterial phase hyperenhancement and washout in the portal venous or delayed phase. However, HCC showing an infiltrative growth pattern might be

Japanese Vp classification	Venous involvement	Cheng's classification
Vp1	Involvement of the segmental branches of PV.	**Type I**
Vp2	Involvement of second order branches	
Vp3	Involvement of first order branches	**Type II**
Vp4	Involvement of the main trunk	**Type III**
	Involvement of SMV	**Type IV**

Table 2.
Japanese VP and Cheng's classification systems for PVTT.

difficult to diagnose as it is usually ill-defined and shows minimal arterial enhancement. The presence of associated malignant thrombus might be the key to diagnosing it [16].

A-VENA non-invasive diagnostic criteria were established by Sherman, C. B., et al. [34]. These criteria depend on the presence of three or more indicators for differentiating PVTT from PVT:

A – alpha-fetoprotein levels more than 1,000 ng/dL

V – venous expansion

E – Enhancement of the thrombus

N – Neovascularity

A – Adjacency to HCC

The extent of PVTT can be assessed by the two most commonly used systems, which are the Japanese VP classification [35, 36] (**Table 2**) and Cheng's classification [37], or the new simplified classification system developed by Xu et al. [38], as described below:

4.1.1 VP classification

The extent of tumor thrombus in the portal vein is divided into four levels in the VP classification (**Figure 2**):

Vp1: The thrombus extends through the segmental branches of the portal vein, distal to the second-order branches.

Vp2: The thrombus extends through the second-order branches.

Vp3: The thrombus extends through the first-order branches of either the right main portal vein or the left main portal vein.

Vp4: The thrombus extends through the main trunk of the portal vein and/or the contralateral branch.

4.1.2 Cheng's classification

In Cheng's classification, there are four grades for thrombus extension:

Type I: The thrombus involves the segmental branches of the portal vein or distal to it (corresponding to Vp1 and Vp2 in the Japanese VP classification).

Type II: The thrombus involves the right or left portal vein (corresponding to Vp3 in the Japanese VP classification).

Type III: The thrombus involves the main portal vein (corresponding to Vp4 in the Japanese VP classification).

Type IV: The thrombus extends to the superior mesenteric vein.

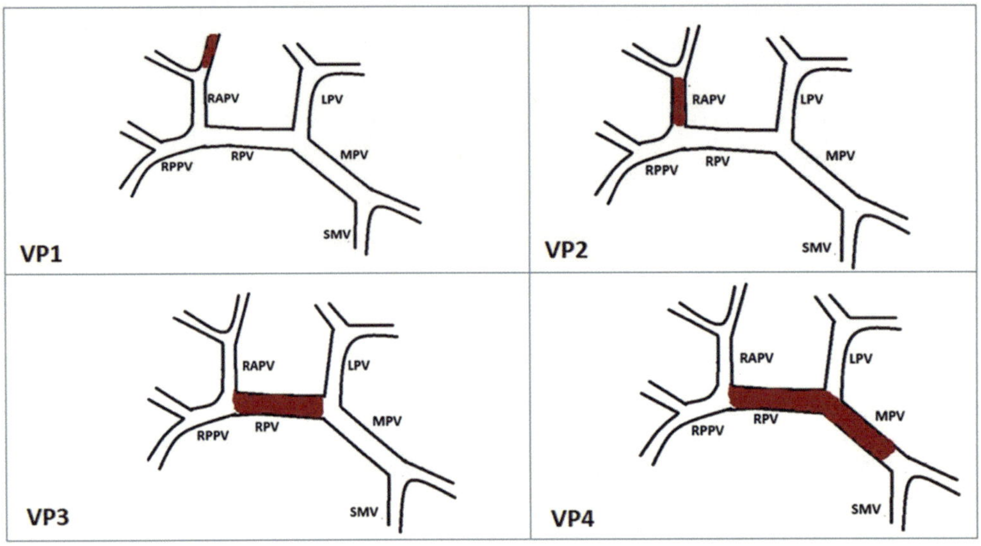

Figure 2.
VP classification system for PVTT.

4.1.3 Xu et al. New classification

They divided PVTT into two groups (**Figure 3**):

Group A: The thrombus involves the main trunk of the portal vein or both the left and right portal veins.

Group B: The thrombus involves only the right or left portal vein.

4.2 Hepatic vein and inferior vena cava invasion

Invasion of hepatic veins (HVTT) in HCC patients is rare compared to PVTT. Invasion of the IVC has been reported to occur in less than 5% of cases, which are considered advanced-stage disease, with therapy limited to only chemotherapy, and survival times not exceeding one year. Extension into the IVC occurs through the invasion of the hepatic veins [39, 40].

A new classification system for hepatic venous invasion was developed by Chen, Z. H., et al. [2] as follows:

Type I: tumor thrombosis involving HV, including microvascular invasion, with two subtypes:

Type Ia: tumor thrombosis extends through the peripheral HV.

Type IB: tumor thrombosis extends through the major HV.

Type II: tumor thrombosis extends through the retrohepatic segment of the inferior vena cava.

Type III: tumor thrombosis extends through the supradiaphragmatic segment of the inferior vena cava with two subtypes (**Figures 4, 5**):

Type IIIa: tumor thrombosis not extending into right atrium.

Type IIIb: tumor thrombosis extending into the right atrium.

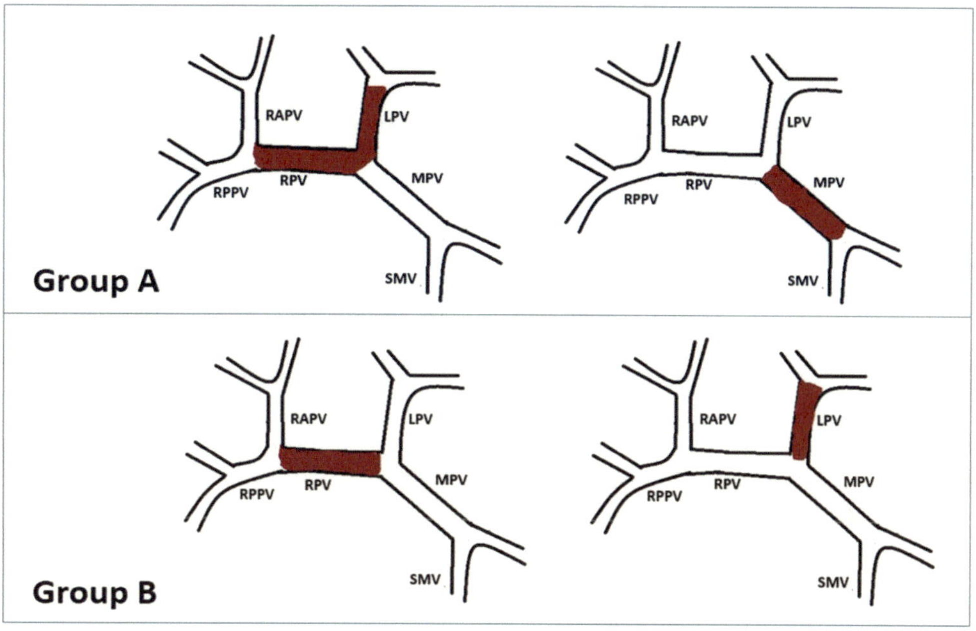

Figure 3.
Xu classification system for PVTT.

5. Hemodynamic changes in portal or hepatic venous invasion

The normal liver has a dual blood supply (70% from the portal vein and 30% from the hepatic artery). The presence of PVTT and HVTT may result in several patterns of hemodynamic changes within the liver in dynamic contrast-enhanced CT [18]. Transient hepatic attenuation differences (THAD) may be associated with venous invasion resulting from arterial phase hyperperfusion [41].

The pathogenic mechanisms mediating THADs are described by Colagrande et al., including:

- Primary arterial inflow in a hyper vascular focal lesion, leading to hyperperfusion of the surrounding parenchyma (siphoning effect).
- Indirectly, by portal hypoperfusion that occurs due to compression or infiltration of the portal vein, thrombosis leading to blockage of a portal branch, or the diversion of flow through an arterioportal shunt. In HCC cases, considerable arteriovenous shunting may occur (**Figure 5**).

Hemodynamic alterations occurring due to PVTT or HVTT are dependent on the size of the shunt. A small portal or hepatic thrombus will not cause significant hemodynamic changes, but large PVTT can significantly diminish portal flow with consequent arterialized perfusion in the distal segment, which may result in a THAD. If the thrombus extends to the IVC, it can lead to congestive hepatopathy by obstructing the liver's venous drainage; if it is larger, it could result in congestion affecting the drainage of the lower limbs and abdominal organs [18].

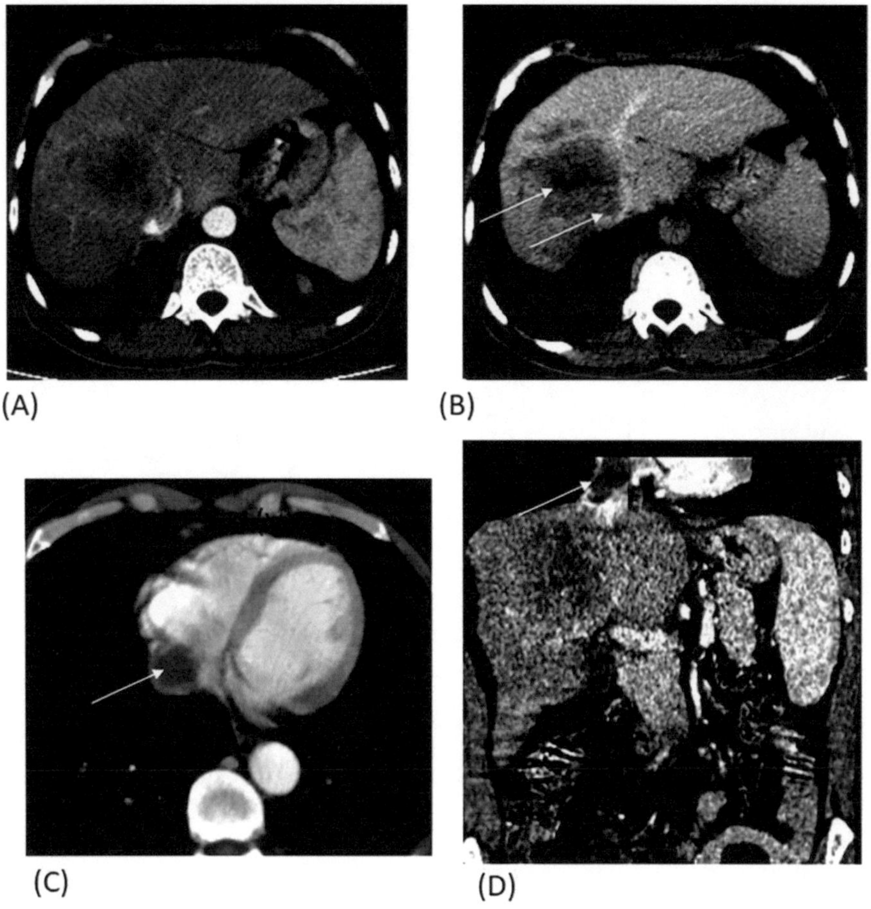

Figure 4.
Axial (a, b, c) and coronal (d) CT images for a case of HCC showing invasion of the right hepatic vein and IVC, extending to its supradiaphragmatic portion.

6. Prognostic factors and staging of vascular invasion in hepatocellular carcinoma

6.1 Prognostic factors in hepatocellular carcinoma with vascular invasion

Involvement of the main portal vein by malignant thrombus causes portal hypertension, with subsequent gastrointestinal bleeding and ascites. PVTT is also a possible cause of multiple intrahepatic tumor seeding and recurrence [42].

Involvement of the inferior vena cava by tumor thrombus and the right atrium can lead to several complications, including secondary Budd–Chiari syndrome, pulmonary embolism, and pulmonary metastases [43].

In addition, it can cause sudden pulmonary embolism, refractory heart failure, and abrupt mortality may occur if the malignant thrombus infiltrates the heart. The prognosis is usually poor, with a reported median survival time of only 2–5 months without treatment [43, 44].

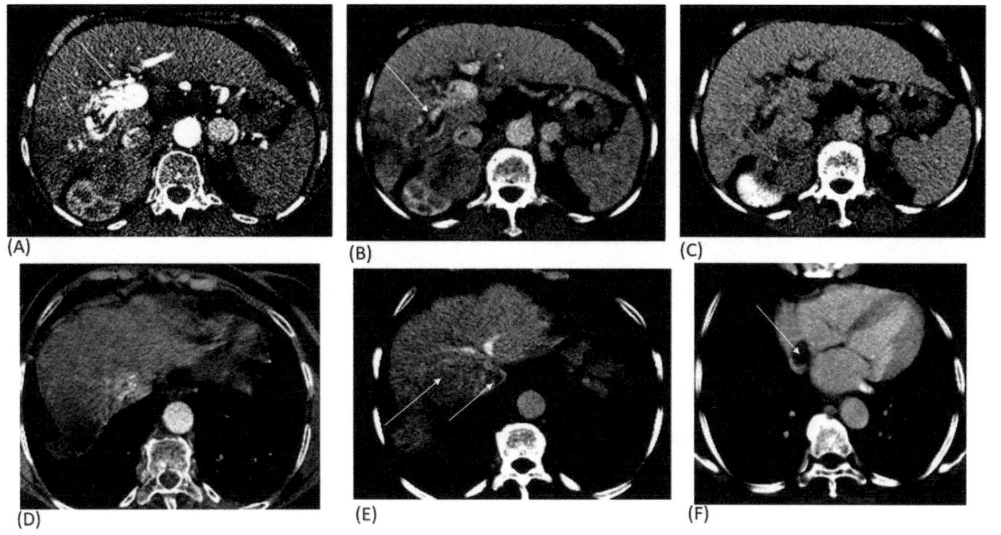

Figure 5.
Axial triphasic study for HCC infiltrative type case showing expansion of the portal vein with early arterial enhancement, denoting an arterioportal shunt (a). Also, there is invasion of the right hepatic vein and the IVC up to the level of the right atrium (arrows in e and f). In this case, there is right adrenal, which is pathologically proven (green arrow).

6.2 Staging Systems

Several staging frameworks are used in HCC, each with distinct strengths and limitations.

The BCLC classification is the most widely adopted globally, linking prognosis with treatment allocation. However, it has been criticized for being overly restrictive; patients with PVTT are considered high stage with recommended systemic therapies only [45].

The Hong Kong Liver Cancer (HKLC) system provides a more aggressive algorithm and has shown superior prognostic stratification, particularly in selected populations with a high prevalence of hepatitis B [46].

The American Joint Committee on Cancer/Union for International Cancer Control (AJCC/UICC) staging system is primarily morphology-based and incorporates vascular invasion, making it valuable for surgical candidates and pathology reporting [10].

7. Causes of missing venous invasion

7.1 Inadequate imaging

Inadequate contrast intake degrades adequate opacification of the venous structures. In addition, single-phase imaging might cause misinterpretation of flow artifacts and distinguishing them from intravenous malignant thrombus; delayed imaging helps in differentiating flow artifacts from actual thrombus by the filling of veins in delayed imaging.

7.2 A similar pattern of malignant thrombus to the primary tumor

As malignant thrombus shows similar features to the primary HCC, the malignant thrombus looks like part of the tumor, and sometimes the venous structure cannot be discriminated separately from the primary tumor, especially if the radiologist forgets to revise the venous structures.

7.3 Forgetting to revise hepatic veins and IVC

The hepatic veins and the IVC are not usually written in templates and are uncommonly invaded in cases of HCC; it is important to search for their patency in each case of HCC.

7.4 Doctor exhaustion and overworking

Doctor exhaustion has a great negative impact on reporting and might be a cause of missing many important findings, such as malignant venous invasion.

8. Conclusion

Hepatocellular carcinoma is the most common malignant tumor with a propensity for venous invasion, mostly involving the portal vein (PVTT) and, less commonly, the hepatic veins and inferior vena cava. Accurate detection and discrimination between bland and malignant thrombus are crucial, as misinterpretation can alter staging, prognosis, and treatment planning. Triphasic CT plays a pivotal role in detecting malignant venous invasion and defining its extent, as the presence of macrovascular invasion usually signifies advanced disease, limiting curative options such as resection or transplantation.

Abbreviations

AFP	Alpha fetoprotein
BCLC	Barcelona Clinic Liver Cancer classification
CT	Computed tomography
DESCT	Dual-energy spectral computed tomography
FDG-PET/CT	Fluorodeoxyglucose positron emission tomography/computed tomography
HCC	Hepatocellular carcinoma
HV	Hepatic vein
HVTT	Hepatic vein tumor thrombus
IVC	Inferior vena cava
MRI	Magnetic resonance imaging
NECT	Non enhanced CT
PVT	Bland portal vein thrombosis
PVTT	Portal vein tumor thrombus
THAD	Transient hepatic attenuation difference

DOI: http://dx.doi.org/10.5772/intechopen.1013466

Conflict of interest

This chapter did not obtain any particular funding from agencies in the public, commercial, or non-profit sectors. The authors declare that there are no conflicts of interest associated with this work.

Author details

Youstina Elamir* and Mai Ashraf Saad Zaghloul
National Cancer Institute, University hospital in Cairo, Cairo, Egypt

*Address all correspondence to: dryousyamir@cu.edu.eg

References

[1] Carr BI. Review of therapies for intermediate and advanced stage hepatocellular carcinoma, not suitable for curative therapies: A rapidly changing landscape HHS Public Access. Hepatoma Research. 2019;**5**:113. DOI: 10.20517/2394-5079.2018.113

[2] Chen ZH, Wang K, Zhang XP, Feng JK, Chai ZT, Guo WX, . . . Cheng SQ. 2020. A new classification for hepatocellular carcinoma with hepatic vein tumor thrombus. Hepatobiliary Surgery and Nutrition. **9** (6):717. DOI: 10.21037/hbsn.2019.10.07

[3] Wang Y, Yuan L, Ge RL, et al. Survival benefit of surgical treatment for hepatocellular carcinoma with inferior vena cava/right atrium tumor thrombus: Results of a retrospective cohort study. Annals of Surgical Oncology. 2013;**20**:914–922

[4] Mizuno S, Kato H, Azumi Y, et al. Total vascular hepatic exclusion for tumor resection: A new approach to the intrathoracic inferior vena cava through the abdominal cavity by cutting the diaphragm vertically without cutting the pericardium. Journal of Hepato-Biliary-Pancreatic Sciences. 2010;**17**:197–202

[5] Piscaglia F, Gianstefani A, Ravaioli M, et al. Criteria for diagnosing benign portal vein thrombosis in the assessment of patients with cirrhosis and hepatocellular carcinoma for liver transplantation. Liver Transplantation. 2010;**16**:658–667

[6] Lee HK, Park SJ, Yi BH, Yeon EK, Kim JH, Hong HS. Portal vein thrombosis: CT features. Abdominal Imaging. 2008;**33**:72–79. DOI: 10.1007/s 00261-007-9200-x

[7] Shah SA, Greig PD, Gallinger S, et al. Factors associated with early recurrence after resection for hepatocellular carcinoma and outcomes. Journal of the American College of Surgeons. 2006;**202**:275–283

[8] Portolani N, Coniglio A, Ghidoni S, et al. Early and late recurrence after liver resection for hepatocellular carcinoma: Prognostic and therapeutic implications. Annals of Surgery. 2006;**243**:229–235

[9] Rohatgi S, Howard SA, Tirumani SH, Ramaiya NH, Krajewski KM. Multimodality imaging of tumour thrombus. Canadian Association of Radiologists Journal. 2015;**66**(2):121–129. DOI: 10.1016/j. carj.2014.11.001

[10] Vauthey JN, Lauwers GY, Esnaola NF, et al. Simplified staging for hepatocellular carcinoma. Journal of Clinical Oncology. 2002;**20**(6):1527–1536. DOI: 10.1200/jco.2002.20.6.1527

[11] Rodriguez-Peralvarez M, Luong TV, Andreana L, Meyer T, Dhillon AP, Burroughs AK. A systematic review of microvascular invasion in hepatocellular carcinoma. Annals of Surgical Oncology. 2013;**20**(1):325–339. DOI: 10.1245/s10434-012-2513-1

[12] Qian LJ, Zhu J, Zhuang ZG, Xia Q, Cheng YF, Li JY, Xu JR. Differentiation of neoplastic from bland macroscopic portal vein thrombi using dual-energy spectral CT imaging: A pilot study. European Radiology. 2012;**22**(10):2178–2185. DOI: 10.1007/s00330-012-2477-3

[13] Buller H, Wouter ten Cate J. Primary venous thromboembolism and

cancer screening. New England Journal of Medicine. 1998;**338**:1221–1222. DOI: 10.1056/nejm199804233381709

[14] Engelbrecht M, Akin O, Dixit D, Schwartz L. Bland and tumor thrombi in abdominal malignancies: Magnetic resonance imaging assessment in a large oncologic patient population. Abdominal Imaging. 2011;**36**:62–68. DOI: 10.1007/s00261-010-9608-6

[15] Khosa F, Otero HJ, Prevedello LM, Rybicki FJ, Di Salvo DN. Imaging presentation of venous thrombosis in patients with cancer. American Journal of Roentgenology. 2010;**194**(4): 1099–1108. DOI: 10.2214/ajr.09.2501

[16] LeGout JD, Bailey RE, Bolan CW, Bowman AW, Chen F, Cernigliaro JG, Alexander LF. Multimodality imaging of abdominopelvic tumors with venous invasion. Radiographics. 2020;**40** (7):2098–2116. DOI: 10.1148/ rg.2020200047

[17] Turun S, Banghua L, Zheng S, Wei Q. Is tumor size a reliable predictor of histopathological characteristics of renal cell carcinoma? Urology Annals. 2012;**4**(1):24–28. DOI: 10.4103/0974-7796.91617

[18] Thompson SM, Wells ML, Andrews JC, Ehman EC, Menias CO, Hallemeier CL, … Venkatesh SK. Venous invasion by hepatic tumors: Imaging appearance and implications for management. 2018; Abdominal Radiology. **43**(8):1947–1967. DOI: 10.1 007/s00261-017-1298-x

[19] Agarwal KK, Shah D, Shah N, Mayank M. 2017. Differentiation of malignant thrombus from bland thrombus of the portal vein in patient with hepatocellular carcinoma on 18F-FDG PET CT. Clinical Nuclear Medicine. **42**(11):e472–e474. DOI: 10.1 097/rlu.0000000000001840

[20] Wu B, Zhang Y, Tan H, Shi H. 2019. Value of 18F-FDG PET/CT in the diagnosis of portal vein tumor thrombus in patients with hepatocellular carcinoma. Abdominal Radiology. **44** (7):2430–2435. DOI: 10.1007/s00261-0 19-01997-2

[21] Khosa F, Otero HJ, Prevedello LM, Rybicki FJ, Di Salvo DN. Imaging presentation of venous thrombosis in patients with cancer. American Journal of Roentgenology. 2010;**194**(4): 1099–1108. DOI: 10.2214/ajr.09.2501

[22] Canellas R, Mehrkhani F, Patino M, Kambadakone A, Sahani D. Characterization of portal vein thrombosis (neoplastic versus bland) on CT images using software-based texture analysis and thrombus density (hounsfield units). American Journal of Roentgenology. 2016;**207**(5):W81–W87. DOI: 10.2214/ajr.15.15928

[23] Ascenti G, Sofia C, Mazziotti S, et al. Dual-energy CT with iodine quantification in distinguishing between bland and neoplastic portal vein thrombosis in patients with hepatocellular carcinoma. Clinical Radiology. 2016;**71**(9):938e1–938e9. DOI: 10.1016/j.crad.2016.05.002

[24] Peng YJ, Dai T, Li D, Liu P, He YQ. Value of dual-energy computed tomography quantitative parameters in differentiating neoplastic from bland portal vein thrombosis. Quantitative Imaging in Medicine and Surgery. 2025;**15**(6):5101. DOI: 10.21037/qims-2 024-2516

[25] Yeh BM, Shepherd JA, Wang ZJ, Teh HS, Hartman RP, Prevrhal S.

Dual-energy and low-kVp CT in the abdomen. American Journal of Roentgenology. 2009;**193**:47–54. DOI: 10.2214/ajr.09.2592

[26] Fletcher JG, Takahashi N, Hartman R, et al. Dual-energy and dual-source CT: Is there a role in the abdomen and pelvis? Radiologic Clinics of North America. 2009;**47**:41–57

[27] Parvey HR, Raval B, Sandler CM. Portal vein thrombosis: Imaging findings. American Journal of Roentgenology. 1994;**162**:77–81. DOI: 10.2214/ajr.162.1.8273695

[28] Llovet JM, Bustamante J, Castells A, Vilana R, Del Carmen Ayuso M, Sala M, et al. Natural history of untreated nonsurgical hepatocellular carcinoma: Rationale for the design and evaluation of therapeutic trials. Hepatology. 1999;**29**(1):62–67. DOI: 10.1002/hep.510290145

[29] Quirk M, Kim YH, Saab S, Lee EW. Management of hepatocellular carcinoma with portal vein thrombosis. World Journal of Gastroenterology. 2015;**21**(12):3462–3471. DOI: 10.3748/wjg.v21.i12.3462

[30] Minagawa M, Makuuchi M. Treatment of hepatocellular carcinoma accompanied by portal vein tumor thrombus. World Journal of Gastroenterology. 2006;**12**(47):7561–7567. DOI: 10.3748/wjg.v12.i47.7561

[31] Sun L, GUAN YS, PAN WM, et al. Positron emission tomography computer tomography in guidance of extra-hepatic hepatocellular carcinoma metastasis management. The World Journal of Gastroenterology. 2007;**13**(40):5413. DOI: 10.3748/wjg.v13.i40.5413

[32] Hennedige T, Venkatesh SK. Advances in computed tomography and magnetic resonance imaging of hepatocellular carcinoma. World Journal of Gastroenterology. 2016;**22**(1):205–220. DOI: 10.3748/wjg.v22.i1.205

[33] Ponziani FR, Zocco MA, Campanale C, Rinninella E, Tortora A, Maurizio LD, et al. Portal vein thrombosis: Insight into physiopathology, diagnosis, and treatment. World Journal of Gastroenterology. 2010;**16**(2):143–155. DOI: 10.3748/wjg.v16.i2.143

[34] Sherman CB, Behr S, Dodge JL, Roberts JP, Yao FY, Mehta N. Distinguishing tumor from bland portal vein thrombus in liver transplant candidates with hepatocellular carcinoma: The A-VENA criteria. Liver Transplantation. 2019;**25**(2):207–216. DOI: 10.1002/lt.25345

[35] Liver Cancer Study Group of Japan. The general rules for the clinical and pathological study of primary liver cancer. The Japanese Journal of Surgery. 1989;**19**:98–129. DOI: 10.1007/BF02471576

[36] Ikai I, Yamamoto Y, Yamamoto N, Terajima H, Hatano E, Shimahara Y, et al. Results of hepatic resection for hepatocellular carcinoma invading major portal and/or hepatic veins. Surgical Oncology Clinics of North America. 2003;**12**(1):65–75. DOI: 10.1016/S1055-3207(02)00082-0

[37] Shuqun C, Mengchao W, Han C, Feng S, Jiahe Y, Guanghui D, et al. Tumor thrombus types influence the prognosis of hepatocellular carcinoma with the tumor thrombi in the portal

vein. Hepato-gastroenterology. 2007;**54**:499–502

[38] Xu JF, Liu XY, Wang S, Wen HX. Surgical treatment for hepatocellular carcinoma with portal vein tumor thrombosis: A novel classification. World Journal of Surgical Oncology. 2015;**13**:1–5. DOI: 10.1186/s12957-015-0493-x

[39] Lee IJ, Chung JW, Kim HC, Yin YH, So YH, Jeon UB, . . . Park JH. Extrahepatic collateral artery supply to the tumor thrombi of hepatocellular carcinoma invading inferior vena cava: The prevalence and determinant factors. Journal of Vascular and Interventional Radiology. 2009;**20** (1):22–29. DOI: 10.1016/j.jvir.2008.09.030

[40] Kokudo T, Hasegawa K, Matsuyama Y, Takayama T, Izumi N, Kadoya M. Liver Cancer Study Group of Japan Liver resection for hepatocellular carcinoma associated with hepatic vein invasion: A Japanese nationwide survey. Hepatology. 2017;**66**(2):510–517. DOI: 10.1002/hep.29225

[41] Colagrande S, Centi N, La Villa G. Villari N Transient hepatic attenuation differences. American Journal of Roentgenology. 2004;**183**(2):459–464. DOI: 10.2214/ajr.183.2.1830459

[42] Tadokoro T, Tani J, Morishita A, Fujita K, Masaki T, Kobara H. The treatment of hepatocellular carcinoma with major vascular invasion. Cancers. 2024;**16**(14):2534. DOI: 10.3390/cancers16142534

[43] Chern MC, Chuang VP, Cheng T, Lin ZH, Lin YM. Transcatheter arterial chemoembolization for advanced hepatocellular carcinoma with inferior vena cava and right atrial tumors. CardioVascular and Interventional Radiology. 2008;**31**:735–744. DOI: 10.1007/s00270-008-9342-4

[44] Le Treut YP, Hardwigsen J, Ananian P, Saisse J, Gregoire E, Richa H, Campan P. Resection of hepatocellular carcinoma with tumor thrombus in the major vasculature. A European case-control series. Journal of Gastrointestinal Surgery. 2006;**10**:855–862. DOI: 10.1016/j.gassur.2005.12.011

[45] Llovet JM, Brú C, Bruix J. Prognosis of hepatocellular carcinoma: The BCLC classification. Seminars in Liver Disease. 1999;**19**(3):329–338. DOI: 10.1055/s-2007-1007122

[46] Yau T, Tang VY, Yao TJ, et al. Development of Hong Kong Liver Cancer staging system. Gastroenterology. 2014;**146**(7): 1691–1700. DOI: 10.1053/j.gastro.2014.02.032

Chapter 5

Computed Tomography in Comprehensive Oncologic Evaluation: Integration with Molecular PET Imaging

Fabio Andrés Sinisterra Solís, Emilly Alejandra Cortés Mancera, Sergio Antonio López Buenrostro and Rocío Del Pilar Cortés Quezada

Abstract

Computed tomography (CT) and positron emission tomography (PET) are pivotal imaging modalities in oncology, each offering unique advantages. CT provides high-resolution anatomical details, enabling precise tumor localization, characterization, and TNM staging. However, its reliance on structural data limits its ability to assess metabolic activity. Conversely, PET, particularly with [^{18}F]-FDG, captures functional and molecular processes, revealing tumor viability and heterogeneity. The integration of these modalities in hybrid PET/CT systems has revolutionized oncologic care by combining anatomic precision with metabolic sensitivity, improving diagnostic accuracy, staging, and therapeutic planning. This chapter explores the technical principles of CT and PET, highlighting advancements such as multidetector CT, dual-energy CT, and photon-counting CT, alongside emerging PET radiopharmaceuticals. It underscores the clinical impact of PET/CT in detecting occult metastases, assessing early treatment response, and differentiating recurrence from post-therapeutic changes. Key applications include guiding radiotherapy planning, where metabolic tumor volume (MTV) delineation enhances precision and reduces toxicity. Limitations, such as false positives from inflammatory FDG uptake or CT's inability to discriminate viable tissue, are also discussed. Ultimately, PET/CT exemplifies precision medicine, enabling tailored oncologic management. Its role in optimizing staging, prognostication, and therapy monitoring underscores its indispensability in modern oncology. Future directions, including novel tracers and AI-driven analysis, promise further advancements in cancer imaging and patient outcomes.

Keywords: computed tomography, PET/CT, oncology, molecular imaging, cancer, diagnostic imaging

1. Introduction

Cancer remains one of the leading causes of morbidity and mortality worldwide [1]. In this context, early detection and comprehensive diagnostic evaluation are fundamental pillars for improving clinical outcomes and overall survival rates [2]. Over the past decades, medical imaging has evolved as a key tool, enabling not only the identification of lesions but also the understanding of their biological behavior, thereby facilitating more personalized and efficient care [3].

Computed tomography (CT) has long been one of the most reliable methods for obtaining precise anatomical images. Thanks to its ability to generate high-resolution multiplanar slices, it has proven accurate in locating, characterizing, and staging various types of solid tumors [4]. Its evolution, from the first single-slice scanners to advanced technologies such as multidetector CT, dual-energy CT, and photon-counting CT, has expanded its diagnostic utility and optimized therapeutic planning [5].

However, conventional CT provides structural information but lacks functional and molecular data on tumor activity. In this regard, positron emission tomography (PET), especially with [^{18}F]-FDG (fluorodeoxyglucose), adds a fundamental metabolic dimension for assessing neoplastic activity, reflecting the biological behavior of cancer. The integration of both modalities into a single hybrid PET/CT study has revolutionized oncologic approaches, improving staging, detection of occult metastases, differentiation between recurrence and post-treatment changes, and evaluation of metabolic response [3, 6], among other less-explored scenarios.

Various studies have shown that PET/CT can modify the treatment plan in up to 35% of cases, depending on the cancer type and oncologic scenario, by detecting lesions not evident in other modalities or redefining tumor extent. Additionally, it has proven useful in different cancer types, including Hodgkin and non-Hodgkin lymphoma, lung, breast, prostate, colorectal, gynecologic, esophageal, pancreatic, and head and neck cancers, as well as in postoperative follow-up and radiotherapy planning. In the latter field, it allows more precise delineation of target volumes, reducing exposure to healthy tissues and increasing therapeutic efficacy [6, 7].

This chapter aims to explore the added value of the diagnostic synergy between CT and molecular PET imaging, highlighting its technical foundations, real clinical impact in various scenarios where patient lives depend on well-founded decisions, and, beyond protocols, how integrating both modalities represents a commitment to precision, personalized medicine, and excellence in oncologic care.

2. Technical principles of computed tomography

2.1 Fundamentals and historical evolution

CT is based on the attenuation of X-rays as they pass through body tissues and the mathematical reconstruction of cross-sectional images from these projections. Unlike conventional radiography, where overlapping structures can limit visualization, CT provides precise anatomical slices using algorithms derived from the Radon transform, published in 1917, and later operationalized by Allan Cormack and Godfrey Hounsfield, who introduced the first clinical scanners in the 1970s [8, 9].

The first devices offered cranial images with low resolution (80x80 pixel matrix) and prolonged acquisition times of up to 7 minutes per slice. However, progressive technological advances led to systems with continuous rotation, multiple detectors, and rapid image reconstruction, laying the groundwork for helical and multidetector tomography [9].

2.2 Current technology: Multidetector CT, dual-energy CT, and photon-counting CT

Multidetector CT (MDCT) has almost entirely replaced single-detector-row systems. It uses two-dimensional detector arrays to acquire multiple slices simultaneously, significantly reducing scan time and improving spatial resolution. This capability is particularly useful in oncology, where evaluating multiple organs in a single scan is crucial for staging and therapeutic planning [9, 10].

Dual-energy CT (DECT) uses two energy levels (typically 80 and 140 kVp) to obtain spectral information about tissue composition. It allows differentiation of materials such as calcium, iodine, and uric acid and generates virtual non-contrast maps. This technique improves lesion detection in the liver, lymph nodes, and bone structures and is particularly promising in thoracic and abdominal oncology [11].

In the newest approach, emerging photon-counting CT technology uses detectors capable of directly counting individual photons passing through the body, rather than converting them into intermediate signals. This modality improves spatial resolution, reduces image noise, and enables more precise tissue characterization. Although still in clinical development, it represents the future of high-definition structural imaging [12].

2.3 Strengths and limitations of CT in oncology

CT has been a cornerstone in cancer patient evaluation due to its high anatomical resolution, fast acquisition, accessibility, and ability to assess multiple systems in a single scan. Its utility in detecting primary masses, regional lymphadenopathy, pulmonary and bone metastases positions it as a fundamental tool in TNM staging (Tumor, Node, Metastasis) and target volume delineation for radiotherapy [13–15].

However, conventional CT is limited by its inability to discriminate tumor viability, as structural changes may not accurately reflect the biological activity of the disease. Thus, it cannot reliably differentiate between active tumor tissue, post-treatment fibrosis, or necrosis, which may affect clinical decision-making in ambiguous scenarios. This limitation has driven its integration with functional techniques like PET, enabling complementary and precise metabolic evaluation [15, 16].

3. Role of computed tomography in oncologic diagnosis and staging

3.1 Tumor detection and anatomic characterization

CT plays a central role in detecting primary and secondary lesions in patients with suspected or confirmed cancer. Thanks to its high spatial resolution and multiplanar capability, it allows precise identification and delineation of solid masses, tissue thickening, lymphadenopathy, infiltration of adjacent structures, and patterns suggestive of disseminated disease [13].

The detailed anatomic characterization provided by CT facilitates differentiation between benign and malignant lesions based on morphology, density, contrast enhancement, presence of necrosis, calcifications, and relationships with vascular or lymphatic structures. In abdominal neoplasms, for example, it enables precise evaluation of peritoneal, hepatic, or retroperitoneal involvement; in the thorax, it is essential for studying pulmonary, mediastinal, and pleural extension [4].

Additionally, its rapid acquisition allows imaging of multiple anatomic regions in a single study, which is key for comprehensive cancer staging and initial therapeutic planning [4].

3.2 CT evaluation in TNM staging

The TNM system, developed by the UICC and AJCC, is the basis for classifying cancer extent. CT is an essential tool for evaluating each of these components:

- **T (Primary tumor):** CT measures tumor size, defines margins, identifies invasion of surrounding tissues (e.g., chest wall, vessels, solid organs), and evaluates structural changes.

- **N (Lymph nodes):** While CT primarily assesses size and morphology, it cannot reliably distinguish between reactive hyperplasia and metastatic involvement. However, nodes larger than 1 cm, rounded, with loss of fatty hilum, or abnormal enhancement may be considered suspicious.

- **M (Distant metastasis):** CT is widely used to detect pulmonary, hepatic, adrenal, peritoneal, and bone metastases, among others. Its utility is enhanced with intravenous contrast and multiphase protocols.

Thus, CT not only enables precise staging but also helps select patients for surgery, chemotherapy, immunotherapy, or radiotherapy, contributing to personalized medicine [17, 18]. Despite advances in new imaging techniques, CT remains pivotal, especially in scenarios such as lung cancer [19].

3.3 Limitations in functional characterization

Despite its strengths, CT has inherent limitations as it relies solely on structural data. Often, neoplastic and inflammatory processes share similar morphologic features, complicating differentiation. Moreover, CT cannot definitively determine whether apparently viable tissue is metabolically active or if residual disease persists post-treatment. These limitations are critical in therapeutic response evaluation, where size reduction does not always correlate with the absence of tumor activity [20].

Therefore, integration with functional techniques like PET allows for more comprehensive characterization by providing metabolic information that complements anatomical imaging and improves diagnostic accuracy [15, 16].

4. Principles of PET imaging

PET is a functional and molecular imaging modality that visualizes, characterizes, and quantifies biochemical and physiological disease processes in real time. Its integration with CT in hybrid PET/CT systems has revolutionized oncologic evaluation by combining PET's metabolic sensitivity with CT's anatomic precision [16].

4.1 Physical and biological fundamentals of [^{18}F]-FDG

As part of the principles of molecular imaging, the use of radiopharmaceuticals is essential – that is, the combination of a radioactive isotope attached to a molecular vehicle, which can be a protein, amino acid, receptor, hormone, etc. There are various PET radiopharmaceuticals available for clinical use, and many more are under investigation, particularly in oncology (**Figure 1**, **Table 1**). However, the most widely used radiopharmaceutical in oncology is [^{18}F]-FDG, a glucose analog labeled with fluorine-18. The radioactive isotope, fluorine-18, is used to chemically

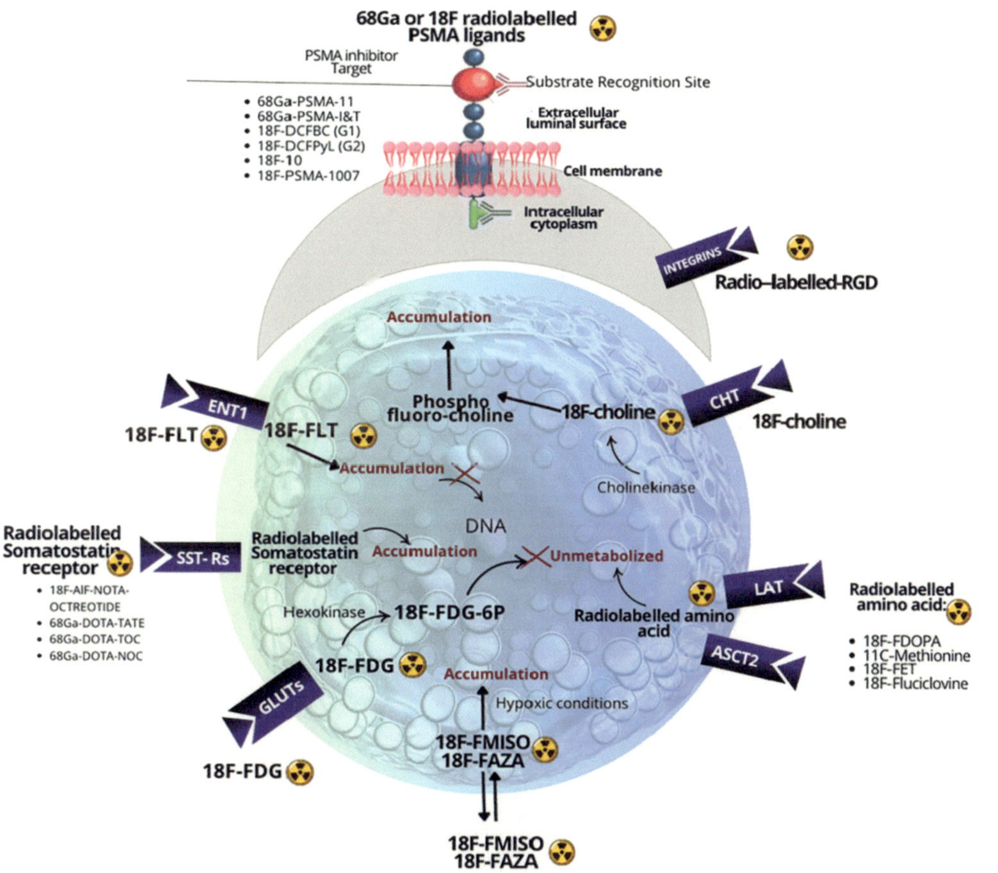

Figure 1.
Main radiopharmaceuticals used in oncology [22]. Used with permission from the publisher.

Radiopharmaceutical	Labeled molecule	Mechanism/Target	Medical indication
^{18}F-FDG	^{18}F-Fluorodeoxyglucose	Evaluates glucose metabolism via GLUT-1 overexpression	Infection/inflammation and oncology
Somatostatin receptor analog: ^{68}Ga-DOTA (e.g., DOTATATE), ^{18}F-NOTA-Octreotide	Octreotide	Increased expression of somatostatin receptors	Neuroendocrine tumors, meningioma
^{68}Ga-PSMA-11	Prostate-specific membrane antigen (PSMA)	Anti-PSMA antibody targets PSMA glycoprotein and evaluates increased tumor vascularity	Prostate cancer
^{18}F-DCFPyL (PSMA)			
^{68}Ga-FAPI	Fibroblast activation protein inhibitor	Targets overexpression of fibroblast activation protein	Tumors with stromal component
^{18}F-FES	Fluoroestradiol	Targets estrogen receptor expression	Estrogen receptor-positive breast cancer
Amino acid transport: ^{11}C-Methionine, ^{18}F-FDOPA, ^{18}F-FET	Amino acids	Increased protein synthesis in the tumor	Braintumors

Table 1.
Commonly used PET radiopharmaceuticals in oncology.

replace a hydroxyl group in glucose. This compound enters cells via glucose transporters (GLUT), especially GLUT-1, and is phosphorylated by hexokinase II. Unlike glucose, phosphorylated FDG becomes trapped inside the cell and does not continue through the glycolytic pathway, thereby allowing visualization of areas with high glucose metabolism, which are typical of many malignant tumors [16, 21].

This principle is based on the Warburg effect, which describes how many tumor cells exhibit increased aerobic glycolysis, consuming large amounts of glucose even in the presence of oxygen. For this reason, [^{18}F]FDG-PET is effective in the detection, staging, assessment of treatment response, and surveillance of a wide variety of tumors, such as lymphoma, lung cancer, colon cancer, breast cancer, and melanoma, among others [16, 21].

4.2 Clinical applications of [^{18}F]-FDG

FDG-PET has become a fundamental tool in oncologic care. Its sensitivity for detecting active neoplastic disease often surpasses that of structural imaging modalities, allowing for:

- Detection of primary lesions that are hidden or not characterized by CT or MRI.
- Early identification of lesions not visible on conventional imaging studies, since physiological changes precede morphological changes (**Figure 2**).
- Evaluation of disease extent (staging and restaging) (**Figure 3**).
- Monitoring of therapeutic response, even before tumor size reduction becomes evident.
- Differentiation between tumor recurrence and post-treatment changes (fibrosis, necrosis).

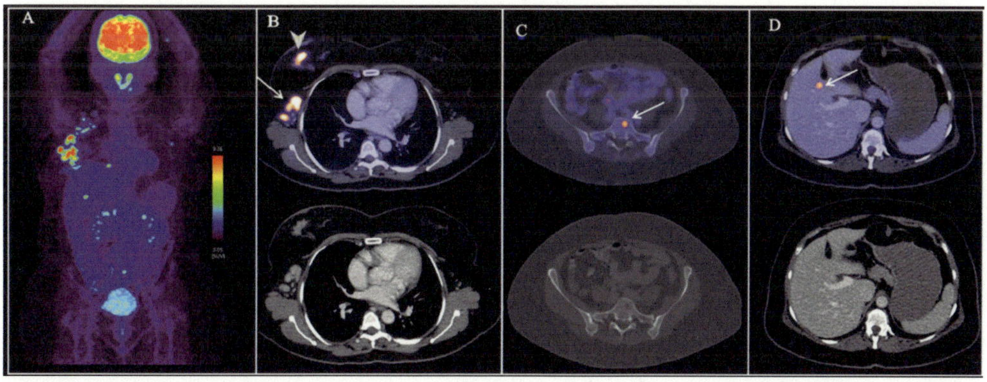

Figure 2.
Staging of a 60-year-old patient diagnosed with metastatic lobular carcinoma of the right breast. a) Maximum intensity projection PET/^{18}F-FDG. b) Breast lesion (arrowhead) and right axillary lymphadenopathy with increased metabolism (arrow). c) Hypermetabolic lytic lesion in the L5 vertebral body (arrow). d) Hepatic lesion without tomographic correlation (arrow).

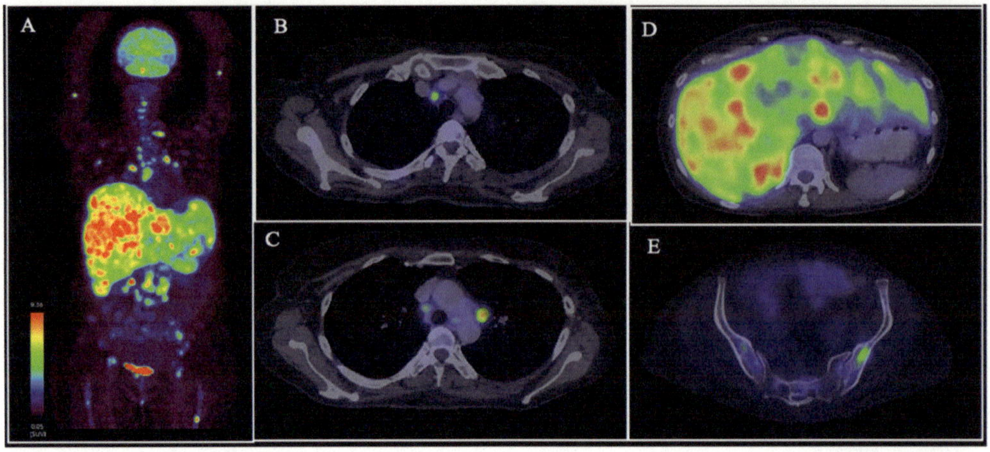

Figure 3.
Restaging of a 48-year-old patient diagnosed with left breast cancer. a) Maximum intensity projection PET/^{18}F-FDG. b) Hypermetabolic right upper paratracheal lymph node. c) Hypermetabolic mediastinal lymph nodes: right lower paratracheal and paraaortic. d) Hypermetabolic hepatic lesions. e) Hypermetabolic lesion in the left iliac bone.

- Detection of distant metastases with greater sensitivity, particularly in the liver, lungs, lymph nodes, bones, and peritoneum.

In addition, the sequential acquisition of PET and CT images allows for the generation of metabolic maps fused with anatomical details. This synergy has increased diagnostic accuracy by approximately 4% to 15%, and confidence in anatomical localization by 30% to 50% [21].

4.3 Limitations of FDG-PET

Despite its high sensitivity, FDG-PET has limitations. FDG is not a tumor-specific tracer; it can accumulate in inflammatory or infectious processes, as well as in tissues with naturally high metabolic activity (such as the brain, myocardium, skeletal muscle, or bone marrow). This accumulation can lead to false positives or complicate the interpretation of certain lesions.

In addition, some slow-growing or low-grade tumors – such as certain prostatic adenocarcinomas, neuroendocrine tumors, or mucinous neoplasms – may exhibit low FDG uptake, resulting in false negatives. Therefore, understanding the clinical and histological context, as well as the limitations of the radiotracer, is essential for accurate interpretation [23].

4.4 Semiquantitative parameters and technical advances

The most commonly used parameter in PET evaluation is the SUV (standard uptake value), which allows for the comparison of tumor uptake relative to the patient's body weight and the administered dose. However, this value can be influenced by multiple technical and physiological factors, such as blood glucose levels, post-injection time, equipment calibration, and reconstruction methods.

Recent advances in PET include improved spatial resolution through digital detectors, time-of-flight (TOF) correction, penalized iterative reconstruction (BSREM), and the development of total-body PET, which enables studies with lower doses and higher sensitivity.

From a technical standpoint, current PET/CT systems use multi-ring detectors with iterative reconstruction and attenuation correction based on CT. Image acquisition is performed in multiple transaxial slices, reconfigured into multiplanar reconstructions (coronal and sagittal), generating thousands of images per study. This complexity has driven the development of advanced algorithms and artificial intelligence tools for analysis and interpretation [24, 25].

New quantitative parameters have recently been developed for use in 18 F-FDG PET/CT imaging, namely metabolic tumor volume (MTV) and total lesion glycolysis (TLG). TLG is calculated by multiplying MTV by the average SUV, and it enables the assessment of both the tumor's metabolic activity and volumetric burden. Its utility lies in predicting disease prognosis and evaluating treatment response more reliably [26, 27].

The ongoing development of new radiotracers – targeting markers such as hormone receptors, integrins, or specific antigens – is expanding the field of nuclear medicine toward precision oncology, where PET not only serves as a diagnostic tool but also guides targeted therapies and evaluates molecular biomarkers in real time [21].

5. Integration of CT and PET: Hybrid PET/CT studies

The integration of CT and PET into a single hybrid system has transformed oncologic imaging. By combining the functional information from PET with the anatomical detail provided by CT, it enables more accurate lesion characterization, significantly enhancing diagnostic performance across multiple oncologic clinical scenarios [28, 29].

5.1 Technical principles of image fusion

Accurate fusion of PET/CT images is achieved through sequential or simultaneous acquisition within a single hybrid device. PET provides functional and metabolic information, while CT defines anatomical relationships with high spatial resolution. Automatic coregistration is facilitated by the sharing of the same field of view and spatial coordinates [28, 29].

There are different methods of image fusion:

- Visual (cognitive) fusion: Based on the specialist's subjective comparison of images.

- Software-based fusion (rigid and deformable registration): Utilizes mathematical algorithms to align anatomical structures.

- Simulation in treatment position: For image-guided radiotherapy, acquisition is performed under conditions identical to those of treatment, minimizing spatial uncertainties.

Advances, such as the use of digital detectors, time-of-flight (TOF) technology, and respiratory motion correction, have significantly improved spatial registration accuracy and image quality [28, 29].

5.2 Advantages of hybrid imaging compared to standalone modalities

The PET/CT combination overcomes the inherent limitations of each technique when used separately.

Its main advantages include:

- Greater diagnostic accuracy: Enables the correlation of functional findings with exact anatomical structures.
- Reduction of unnecessary studies: By integrating two modalities into a single session.
- Shorter examination time: Optimizes patient workflow.
- Improved therapeutic planning: Provides metabolic data for radiotherapy, surgery, or follow-up [28, 29].

Clinical studies have shown improvements in staging, changes in therapeutic approaches in over 25% of cases, and a higher detection rate of metastases compared to CT alone [30].

5.3 Impact on oncologic decision-making

5.3.1 Changes in staging or restaging

PET/CT has demonstrated superiority over conventional imaging in the staging of cancers such as lung, esophageal, colorectal, and lymphoma. Its ability to detect occult disease (nodal or distant) allows for the reclassification of the clinical stage in up to 30% of patients, directly impacting treatment selection [30, 31] (**Figure 4**).

5.3.2 Detection of occult metastases

Thanks to its high sensitivity, PET/CT can identify metastases that are not visible on CT, especially in bone marrow, small lymph nodes, or peritoneal structures. This is particularly useful in tumors such as melanoma, breast cancer, prostate cancer, or head and neck cancer, where it may help avoid unnecessary invasive procedures [32] (**Figure 5**).

5.3.3 Early metabolic response assessment

PET/CT enables early evaluation of therapeutic efficacy before morphological changes become evident. This is possible through the quantification of tumor metabolism (SUV) and the application of criteria such as PERCIST. In contrast to RECIST, which focuses on size, PERCIST detects functional changes that better predict survival and prognosis [33] (**Table 2**).

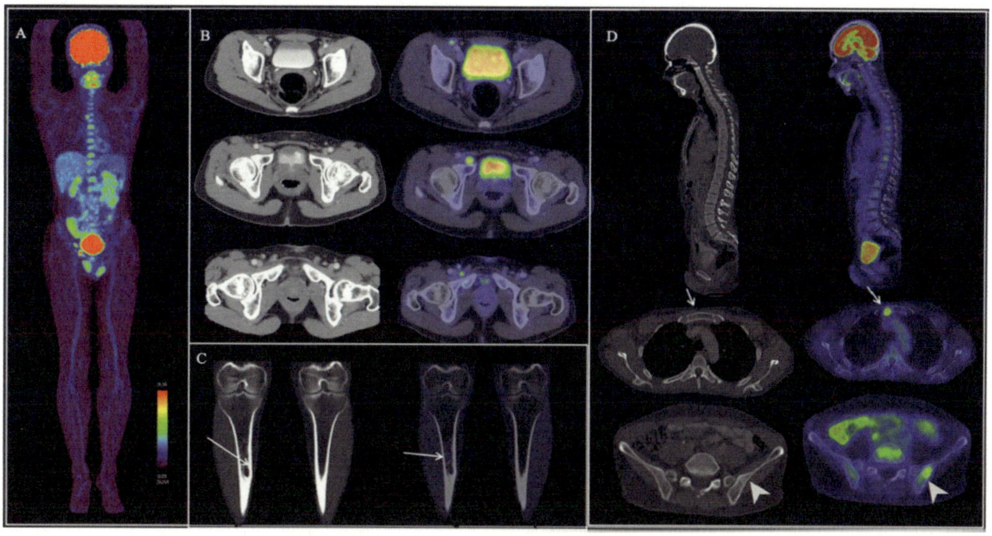

Figure 4.
PET/CT performed to evaluate a primary lesion, with findings related to another condition (lymphoproliferative), and no evidence of neoplastic activity from the primary under investigation. Male patient, 42 year sold, with a history fright tibial enchondroma since 2014. A diagnostic protocol was initiated on 06/05/2025 with MRI reporting a proximal diaphyseal image of the right tibia, suggesting a possible diagnosis of enchondroma with post surgical changes; low-grade chondrosarcoma was considered for exclusion. a) Maximum intensity projection PET/18 F-FDG. b) Adenopathies in the right external iliac and inguinofemoral chains. c) Bone lesion in the proximal third of the right tibia, without aggressive features, consistent with the prior diagnosis of enchondroma (arrows). d) Increased metabolism in the bone marrow of the appendicular skeleton with a heterogeneous pattern and focal areas, some associated with subtle density changes, notably in the sternal manubrium (arrows) and left iliac bone (arrowhead).

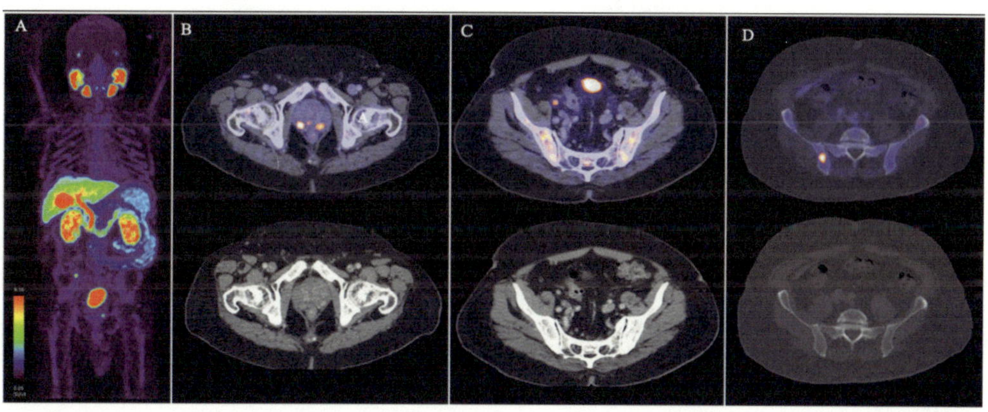

Figure 5.
Staging of prostate adenocarcinoma in a 65-year-old patient with gleason score 4 + 4 = 8 and PSA 88 ng/ml. a) Maximum intensity projection PET/CT PSMA. b) Top row: PET/CT showing areas of radiotracer uptake in the prostate. Bottom row: intraprostatic lesions not defined on CT. c) Top row: PET/CT showing radiotracer uptake in a right iliac lymph node. Bottom row: right iliac lymph node. d) Top row: PET/CT showing focal radiotracer uptake in the right iliac bone. Bottom row: no evidence of lesions on CT.

For example, in the case of hematologic malignancies – primarily Hodgkin and non-Hodgkin lymphoma – 18F-FDG PET/CT is a fundamental tool for evaluating treatment response. The Lugano 2014 guidelines formally incorporate 18F-FDG

CRITERIA	RECIST 1.1	PERCIST
Imaging	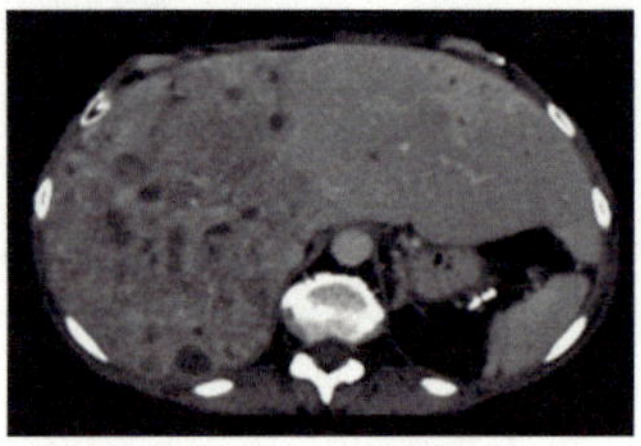	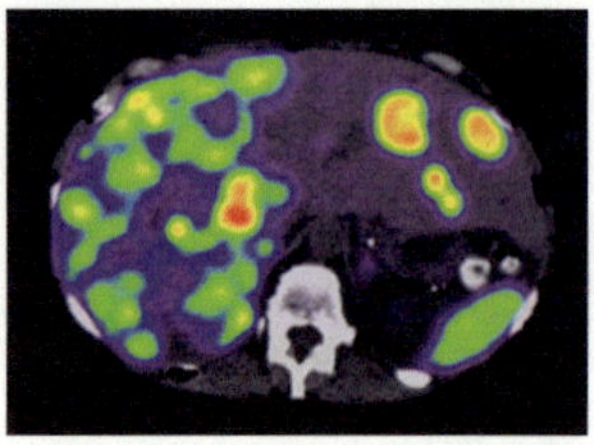
Complete response (CR)	Disappearance of all lesions No evidence of new lesions	Disappearance of all metabolically active lesions
Partial response (PR)Partial response (PR)	30% decrease in the sum of diameters of target lesions	30% decrease and a reduction of 0.8 units in SUL peak between the most intense lesion before and after treatment (not necessarily the same lesion).
Progressive disease (PD)	20% increase in the sum of diameters of target lesions	30% increase and 0.8 units in SUL peak, or new lesions, or 75% increase in total lesionglycolysis
Stable disease (SD)	Neither partial response nor progressive disease	Neither partial response nor progressive disease

Table 2.
Most commonly used response criteria in oncology.

PET/CT for staging and response assessment in FDG-avid lymphomas. The Deauville Scale (5-point) is also used to interpret visual metabolic uptake, comparing it to the mediastinum and liver (scores 1–5 or X) [34, 35] (**Table 3**, **Figure 6**).

5.3.4 Precise radiotherapy planning

In Radiation oncology, PET/CT enables:

- More precise delineation of active tumor volume (metabolic tumor volume, MTV).
- Identification of heterogeneous regions within the tumor that may benefit from focal dose escalation strategies (dose painting).

Deauville score	General interpretation (CMR, PMR, etc.)
1	No abnormal uptake → Complete metabolic response (CMR)
2	Uptake ≤ mediastinum → Complete metabolic response (CMR)
3	Uptake > mediastinum but ≤ liver → Complete metabolic response (CMR), depending on clinical context
4	Moderately higher than liver → Partial metabolic response (PMR) or metabolic progression*
5	Markedly higher uptake or new lesions → Metabolic progression

Table 3.
Response Assessment in Lymphoma.

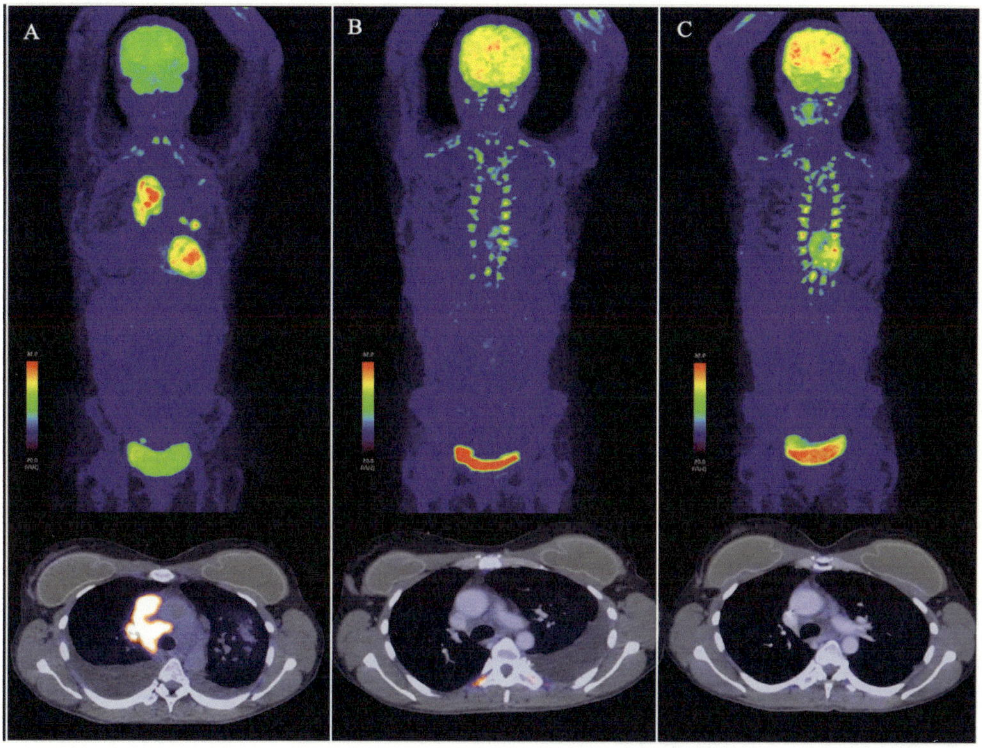

Figure 6.
Response assessment in a patient diagnosed with large b-cell non-hodgkin lymphoma. a) Baseline study: maximum intensity projection PET/18F-FDG showing evidence of mediastinal lymphadenopathy. b) Interim study after 4 cycles of chemotherapy: decreased metabolic activity in mediastinal lymphadenopathy. Deauville score 2. c) End-of treatment study: No evidence of hypermetabolic lesions. Deauville score 1, indicating complete metabolic response.

- Reduced toxicity by avoiding the irradiation of uninvolved healthy tissue.
- Respiratory-synchronized acquisition (gating) is used to minimize blurring in mobile tumors, such as those found in the lungs.

Its implementation enhances the efficacy and safety of radiotherapy, with an increasingly adaptive and personalized approach [31, 32]

6. Conclusions

For many years, the imaging-based diagnostic approach in oncology has been complex. Computed tomography (CT) has played a fundamental role in the initial evaluation due to its accessibility and relatively low cost. However, it presents certain limitations, making it necessary to complement it with functional, metabolic, or molecular studies such as PET, resulting in a hybrid PET/CT scan that provides both functional and anatomical information in a single examination. PET/CT is crucial for staging, assessing treatment response, prognostic evaluation, detecting recurrence, and therapeutic planning. It has become an essential tool in precision medicine. Through the use of various radiopharmaceuticals, PET/CT enables the identification of different metabolic and molecular pathways of the tumor. When applied appropriately and in the correct clinical context, it optimizes decision-making and improves prognosis for cancer patients.

Acknowledgments

The authors gratefully acknowledge the support provided by the medical and academic institutions that contributed to the development of this chapter. Special thanks are extended to the colleagues and professionals whose insightful feedback helped refine the clinical perspectives presented herein. The authors also recognize the invaluable contributions of the technical teams responsible for the acquisition and processing of imaging data. Their expertise and dedication were instrumental in enhancing the quality and depth of this work.

Conflict of interest

The authors declare that there are no conflicts of interest related to this work.

Appendices and nomenclature

PET	Positron emission tomography
CT	Computed tomography
PET/CT	Positron emission tomography/computed tomography
FDG	Fluorodeoxyglucose
PSMA	Prostate specific membrane antigen
SUV	Standardized uptake value
TLG	Total lesion glycolysis
MTV	Metabolic tumor volume

Author details

Fabio Andrés Sinisterra Solís[1*], Emilly Alejandra Cortés Mancera[2], Sergio Antonio López Buenrostro[3] and Rocío Del Pilar Cortés Quezada[4]

1 Molecular Imaging PET/CT Unit, Salud Digna, Mexico City, Mexico

2 Department of Nuclear Medicine and PET/CT, Hospital Ángeles Lomas, Mexico City, Mexico

3 Clinical Pathology and Imaging Unit, Guadalajara, Mexico

4 National Institute of Nutrition and Medical Sciences “Salvador Zubirán”, Mexico City, Mexico

*Address all correspondence to: Fabiosinisterra128@gmail.com

References

[1] Schwartz SM. Epidemiology of cancer. Clinical Chemistry. 2024;**70**(1):140–9

[2] Crosby D, Bhatia S, Brindle KM, Coussens LM, Dive C, Emberton M, Esener S, Fitzgerald RC, Gambhir SS, Kuhn P, Rebbeck TR. Early detection of cancer. Science. 2022;**375**(6586): eaay9040

[3] Visioni A, Kim J. Positron emission tomography for benign and malignant disease. The Surgical Clinics of North America. 2011;**91**(1):249

[4] Bansal A, Dhamija E, Chandrashekhara SH, Sahoo RK. Role of CT in the detection and management of cancer related complications: A study of 599 patients. Ecancermedicalscience. 2023;**17**:1529

[5] Stański M, Michałowska I, Lemanowicz A, Karmelita-Katulska K, Ratajczak P, Sławińska A, Serafin Z. Dual-energy and photon-counting computed tomography in vascular applications—technical background and post-processing techniques. Diagnostics. 2024;**14**(12):1223

[6] Collins CD. PET/CT in oncology: For which tumours is it the reference standard? Cancer Imaging. 2007;**7**(Special issue A):S77–S87

[7] Vijayakumar S, Yang J, Nittala MR, Velazquez AE, Huddleston BL, Rugnath NA, Adari N, Yajurvedi AK, Komanduri A, Yang CC, Duggar WN. Changing role of PET/CT in cancer care with a focus on radiotherapy. Cureus. 2022;**14**(12): e32964

[8] Jung H. Basic physical principles and clinical applications of computed tomography. Progress in Medical Physics. 2021;**32**(1):1–7

[9] Seeram E. Computed tomography: Physical principles and recent technical advances. Journal of Medical Imaging and Radiation Sciences. 2010;**41**(2):87–109

[10] Eltatawy DN, Elsharawy FA, Elbarbary AA, Elsheikh RG, Badawy ME. Multi-detector computed tomography (MDCT) as a diagnostic tool in assessment of thoracic aortic anomalies in pediatric patients. Egyptian Journal of Radiology and Nuclear Medicine. 2021;**52**(1):39

[11] Aran S, Daftari Besheli L, Karcaaltincaba M, Gupta R, Flores EJ, Abujudeh HH. Applications of dual-energy CT in emergency radiology. American Journal of Roentgenology. 2014;**202**(4):W314–W324

[12] Greffier J, Viry A, Robert A, Khorsi M, Si-Mohamed S. Photon-counting CT systems: A technical review of current clinical possibilities. Diagnostic and Interventional Imaging. 2025;**106**(2):53–59

[13] Liguori C, Frauenfelder G, Massaroni C, Saccomandi P, Giurazza F, Pitocco F, Marano R, Schena E. Emerging clinical applications of computed tomography. Medical Devices: Evidence and Research. 2015;**5**:265–278

[14] Rema P, John ER, Samabasivan S, Prahladan A, George P, Ranjith JS,

Thomas S. Evaluation of computed tomography scan and CA 125 response in predicting operability in advanced ovarian cancer and assessing survival outcome in interval cytoreductive surgery. Indian Journal of Surgical Oncology. 2019;**10**(3):426–434

[15] Debbi K, Witweyer S, Bennassi A, Boukhobza C, Fonteneau G, To NH, Coraggio G, Ksouri W, Grellier N, Cherif MA, Loganadane G. Computed tomography (CT)-scan planning in radiation oncology: Prospective evaluation of the "mini-CT-scan" procedure prior to a routinely immediate planning CT-scan practice. Results of the OPTIMAL Study. Advances in Radiation Oncology. 2025;**16**:101808

[16] Griffeth LK. Use of PET/CT scanning in cancer patients: Technical and practical considerations. InBaylor University Medical Center Proceedings. 2005;**18**(4):321–330

[17] Modini C, Passariello R, Iascone C, Cicconetti F, Simonetti G, Zerilli M, Tirindelli-Danesi D, Stipa S. TNM staging in lung cancer: Role of computed tomography. The Journal of Thoracic and Cardiovascular Surgery. 1982;**84**(4):569–574

[18] Duan X, Zhao Q, Li F. Association of CT features with TNM stage and pathology of patients with rectal cancer and their significance in evaluation of efficacy and prognosis. Journal of B.U. ON. : Official Journal of the Balkan Union of Oncology. 2020;**25**:1430–1435

[19] Asamura H, Yotsukura M, Rami-Porta R, Rusch VW. Updates on the Version 9 American Joint Committee on Cancer Staging System for Lung Cancer. Annals of Surgical Oncology. 2025;**32**(7):4569–4571

[20] Czernin J, Allen-Auerbach M, Nathanson D, Herrmann K. PET/CT in Oncology: Current Status and Perspectives. Current Radiology Reports. 2013;**1**(3):177–190. DOI: 10.1007/s40134-013-0016-x

[21] Franquet E, Park H. Molecular imaging in oncology: Common PET/CT radiopharmaceuticals and applications. European Journal of Radiology Open. 2022;**9**:100455

[22] Moreau A, Febvey O, Mognetti T, Frappaz D, Kryza D. Contribution of different positron emission tomography tracers in glioma management: Focus on glioblastoma. Frontiers in Oncology. 2019;**9**:1134. DOI: 10.3389/fonc.2019.01134

[23] Smith CS, Teruya-Feldstein J, Caravelli JF, Yeung HW. False-positive findings on 18F-FDG PET/CT: Differentiation of hibernoma and malignant fatty tumor on the basis of fluctuating standardized uptake values. American Journal of Roentgenology. 2008;**190**(4):1091–1096

[24] Meikle SR, Sossi V, Roncali E, Cherry SR, Banati R, Mankoff D, Jones T, James M, Sutcliffe J, Ouyang J, Petibon Y. Quantitative PET in the 2020s: A roadmap. Physics in Medicine & Biology. 2021;**66**(6):06RM01

[25] Kim SH, Song BI, Kim HW, Won KS. Comparison of image quality and semi-quantitative measurements with digital PET/CT and standard PET/CT from different vendors. Nuclear Medicine and Molecular Imaging. 2020;**54**(5):233–240

[26] Wen W, Piao Y, Xu D, Li X. Prognostic value of MTV and TLG of 18F-FDG PET in patients with stage I and II non-small-cell lung cancer: A

meta-analysis. Contrast Media Mol. Imaging. 2021;**2021**:7528971. DOI: 10.1155/2021/7528971

[27] Wu TH, Liang CH, Wu JK, Lien CY, Yang BH, Huang YH, Lee JJ. Integration of PET-CT and cone-beam CT for image-guided radiotherapy with high image quality and registration accuracy. Journal of Instrumentation. 2009;**4**(07)

[28] Zaidi H, Montandon ML, Alavi A. The clinical role of fusion imaging using PET, CT, and MR imaging. PET Clinics. 2008;**3**(3):275–291

[29] Beyer T, Townsend DW, Czernin J, Freudenberg LS. The future of hybrid imaging—part 2: PET/CT. Insights into Imaging. 2011;**2**(3):225–234

[30] Engel R, Kudura K, Antwi K, Denhaerynck K, Steinemann D, Wullschleger S, Müller B, Bolli M, Torney MV. Diagnostic accuracy and treatment benefit of PET/CT in staging of colorectal cancer compared to conventional imaging. Surgical Oncology. 2024;**57**:102151

[31] Hicks RJ, Ware RE, Lau EW. PET/CT: Will it change the way that we use CT in cancer imaging? Cancer Imaging. 2006;**6**(Special Issue A):S52–S62

[32] Guedj D, Neveü S, Becker M, Mermod M. FDG PET-CT for the detection of occult nodal metastases in head and neck cancer: A systematic review and Meta-Analysis. Cancers. 2024;**16**(17):2954

[33] Puranik AD, Purandare NC, Shah S, Agrawal A, Rangarajan V. Role of FDG PET/CT in assessing response to targeted therapy in metastatic lung cancers: Morphological versus metabolic criteria. Indian Journal of Nuclear Medicine. 2015;**30**(1):21–25

[34] Van Heertum RL, Scarimbolo R, Wolodzko JG, Klencke B, Messmann R, Tunc F, Sokol L, Agarwal R, Strafaci JA, O'Neal M. Lugano 2014 criteria for assessing FDG-PET/CT in lymphoma: An operational approach for clinical trials. Drug Design, Development and Therapy. 2017;**11**:1719–1728. DOI: 10.2147/DDDT.S136988

[35] Trotter J, Pantel AR, Teo BK, Escorcia FE, Li T, Pryma DA, Taunk NK. Positron emission tomography (PET)/computed tomography (CT) imaging in radiation therapy treatment planning: A review of PET imaging tracers and methods to incorporate PET/CT. Advances in Radiation Oncology. 2023;**8**(5):101212